Pauline

Removing the Sting

How Faith, Family and Friends
are helping one woman
face the many challenges
of Parkinson's disease.

A powerful story of God's love and guidance in difficult times.

Pauline J. Neck

Sunrise graphic and photo layouts by Lyn E. Ayre (www.ayresdigitaldoodlings.com)

Cover photo by Elliot Neck. Cates Park photo by David Carr.

All poetry and verse appearing in this book was written by the author between April 1984 and January 2002.

This book is based on the author's personal experience and research as a layperson and is provided as a means of inspiration and encouragement. The spiritual journey is shared in the hope it will comfort those going through similar circumstances.

Readers are advised always to seek the services of competent medical professionals in medical, emotional or other health-related matters.

National Library of Canada Cataloguing in Publication Data
Neck, Pauline J. (Pauline Jane), 1945-
Removing the sting
ISBN 1-55369-223-3
1. Parkinson's disease—Patients—Canada—Biography.
I. Title.
RC382.N42 2002 362.1'96833'0092 C2002-900665-1

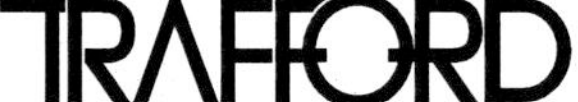

PRINTED IN CANADA

This book was published *on-demand* in cooperation with Trafford Publishing.
On-demand publishing is a unique process and service of making a book available for retail sale to the public taking advantage of on-demand manufacturing and Internet marketing. **On-demand publishing** includes promotions, retail sales, manufacturing, order fulfilment, accounting and collecting royalties on behalf of the author.

Suite 6E, 2333 Government St., Victoria, B.C. V8T 4P4, CANADA
Phone 250-383-6864 Toll-free 1-888-232-4444 (Canada & US)
Fax 250-383-6804 E-mail sales@trafford.com
Web site www.trafford.com TRAFFORD PUBLISHING IS A DIVISION OF TRAFFORD HOLDINGS LTD.
Trafford Catalogue #02-0036 www.trafford.com/robots/02-0036.html

10 9 8 7 6 5 4 3 2

Table of Contents

Acknowledgements

I sincerely thank the following people for helping me write *Removing the Sting*:

- Every member of my family for wholeheartedly supporting this project. The loving encouragement you provided helped me every step of the way. I thank God for you all.

- My dear friends for their many acts of kindness and generosity. Also their infinite patience while I hibernated to complete this book.

- The Coquitlam Alliance Church home team and Maple Ridge Alliance Church family for their loving kindness and prayer support.

- The members of *Women and Words* writing group, without whose encouragement I would never have dared to write at all.

- The Maple Ridge Parkinson's Support Group and Sandy & friends at PLWP (**P**eople **L**iving **W**ith **P**arkinson's) for their kind acceptance, friendship and words of wisdom.

- The incredibly talented people who helped with editing this manuscript: Norman B. Rohrer (Christian Writers Guild), Lenora Vakenti, Ann Lindsay, Carmen Wright, Michaela Wahlers, Margaret Johnson, Donna Morrow, Sharon Corrin, Almut Pfeifer, Doreen Tan, Lois Bird, Beryl Atherton and many other friends and relatives who read sample chapters and gave much valued advice.

- Special thanks to my dear friend and writing mentor, Lyn Ayre, for her editing expertise, knowledge of computer programs, assistance in getting the manuscript ready for printing and also for her considerable talent in scanning and displaying photographs.

- Most importantly, I wish to acknowledge the love and mercy of God, who created in me the enthusiasm to write. Praise the Lord! To Him be all glory and honour!

This book is lovingly dedicated to
my grandchildren Hayley and Maxwell
—two of life's greatest treasures.

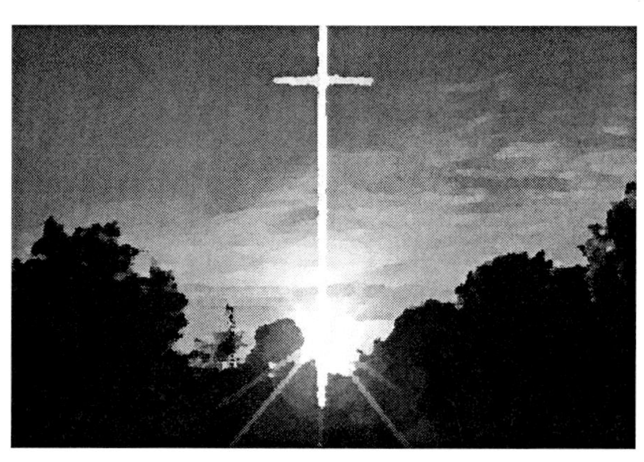

Every morning is a new beginning,
fresh steps to be taken with confidence.
Let us be guided by God's love for us,
so that, in turn, we may guide others
by showing our love for them.

Introduction

An estimated 100,000 Canadians, 120,000 people in the UK, and more than one million Americans are battling Parkinson's disease. Worldwide, the disease afflicts more than four million. Add spouses, care-givers, family and friends and the number of people who are impacted by this debilitating affliction quickly swells to the multi-millions.

Removing the Sting is a true story of how faith in God, a loving family and caring friends are helping me fight against this insidious disease. It is also a descriptive mosaic of the special people in my life, who have helped prepare and strengthen me for the adversity I now face.

I never dreamed I would one day have something in common with former U.S. Attorney General Janet Reno, world renowned evangelist Billy Graham or famous actor Michael J. Fox. The common bond we share is the daily battle of living with a neurological disorder that strikes celebrities and ordinary people alike. Parkinson's disease is certainly no respecter of persons!

My own diagnosis was a great shock, but it also brought a certain feeling of relief. At least I had a name for my health problems and finally knew why I felt so tired.

Life is different now. It takes a little longer to gather my thoughts. Walking is slow and unsteady. Muscles are stiff and painful much of the time. So I try to focus on enjoyable activities, such as reading, writing and visiting with family and friends. Instead of wondering *why*, I strive to count my blessings and maintain a positive attitude (this is a daily, sometimes hourly challenge).

Stress and Parkinson's definitely don't mix so I work hard to *maintain my cool!*

Now content with my life as mother, grandmother,

sister, aunt and friend, I have recently embraced a new family of PLWP (**P**eople **L**iving **W**ith **P**arkinson's). I feel accepted by this amazing group of people who totally understand everything I'm going through. Chatting via the Internet to my new friends at *Sandy's Parkie Porch* has opened up a whole new world of communication with other Parkinsonians. I have also grown to appreciate the members of the Maple Ridge, B.C. Parkinson's Support Group—finding them to be some of the kindest, most courageous people I have ever met.

One of the many truths I have learned while writing this book is... *If one person's adversity can be used to bring a blessing, however small, to another human being, then that particular misfortune has lost its power; it has not won. A soothing balm has been applied to the situation, bringing peace and a renewed sense of purpose.*

> In the words of the Apostle Paul,
> "Therefore we do not lose heart. Though outwardly we are wasting away, yet inwardly we are being renewed day by day. For our light and momentary troubles are achieving for us an eternal glory that far outweighs them all. So we fix our eyes not on what is seen, but on what is unseen. For what is seen is temporary, but what is unseen is eternal."
>
> *~2 Corinthians 4:16 & 17*

When it comes to the realm of the human spirit, I have drawn a line in the sand and will not allow Parkinson's disease to enter. The battle is on...

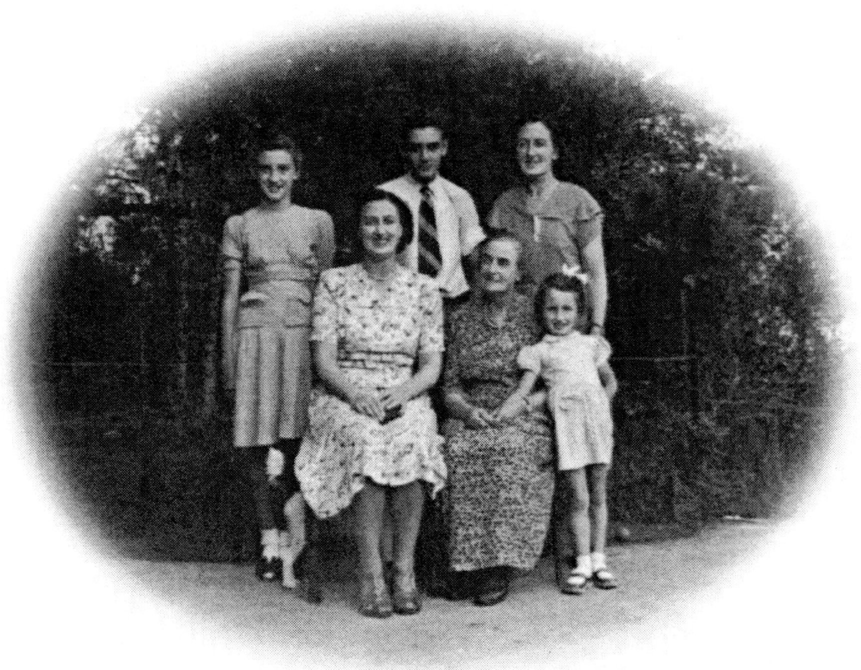

A 1949 family portrait taken by Grandpa Raines in the back yard of our house in Christchurch, England. Standing (L-R) Pat, David, Mummy. Seated (L-R) Auntie Bee, Grandma Raines, with Pauline.

CHAPTER ONE

Survival of the Weakest

My grace is sufficient for you,
for my power is made perfect in weakness.
~2 Corinthians 12:9

I have a hazy childhood memory of snuggling close to my mother in a big arm chair in the living room of our house in Christchurch, England. We are listening to a BBC radio program for children *Listen With Mother*. The volume is turned low because she has a headache.

Some days I concentrate on this memory so hard, my brain hurts. Like a treasure locked away in a vault I take it out and reexamine it, trying with everything in me to discover some other visual record of my mother—her face, her hair, the feel of her hands, but there is nothing else—just the radio, the chair and the sure knowledge that I'm sitting beside her.

Another of my fondest childhood recollections is posing for photographs. Grandpa Raines loved taking pictures of the family and especially us grandkids. He had his own darkroom and we provided him with endless opportunities to practise his hobby. As the undisputed *head* of our family, he was extremely proud of his three daughters—Dorothy, Cecilia (my mother) and Bertha (Auntie Bee).

The oval family portrait shown at the beginning of this chapter is particularly revealing. It was taken in the back garden of our home in Christchurch. On careful study, it shows clearly my brother's teenage good looks, my sister's approaching womanhood and Grandma's regal bearing. Auntie Bee's strength and vitality shine brightly, compared to my mother's gradual fading into illness. As the youngest member of the group, I can see my childlike innocence as I lean against Grandma and place my hand in her lap. The dog obviously wasn't cooperating, as only his back legs and tail are showing.

If a picture is worth a thousand words—this precious photograph taken by Grandpa Raines in 1949, to me is worth a million!

~

Born in 1945, at the end of World War II, I was labeled a *Peace Baby*. As an infant, I was baptized *Pauline Jane Elizabeth Johnson* at Saint Saviour's Church in Bournemouth, Hampshire.[1] Like many other girls born in that era, I had the name Elizabeth added to my first and second names in honour of England's lovely young princess. In 1950, England was still struggling valiantly to recover from the ravages of the Second World War. Many foods were in short supply. As a young girl I purchased candy with stamps from my ration book. There were few luxuries. Daily life was made a little easier when neighbours helped each other.

Our modest semi-detached home was situated a good way back from the street. To enter the property we had to

---

[1] Bournemouth and Christchurch were incorporated into the County of Dorset on April 1, 1974.

walk along a narrow hedge-lined path. My sister hated this pathway, especially after dark when every shadow looked sinister or if spider webs brushed against her face. She was always very relieved to reach the safety of the house.

We did not have electric lights. Each evening Dad lit the gas lamps in our home. As they sputtered and hissed, the dim light cast eerie shadows on the walls, causing all sorts of scary images to appear. Even a bowl of warm bread and milk and the reading of Mother Goose nursery rhymes could not erase the imaginary ghosts and goblins that seemed to creep toward my bed as I tried to fall asleep.

In July 1950, our mother was scheduled for tests at a local hospital. My sister Pat remembers waiting at the bus stop early in the morning and hastily retrieving Mummy's birthday cards from the postman just before the four of us (Mummy, Daddy, Pat and I) got on the bus. I have no recollection of this event, but according to Pat, on arrival at Boscombe Hospital, we said our goodbyes to Mummy at the entrance to the ward. In those days, children were not permitted to enter hospital rooms.

On another occasion my brother, sister and I waved up at Mummy from the street below her hospital window. She seemed very far away.

Two weeks later our mother was transferred to the Atkinson Morley Neurological Hospital in London, where she underwent surgery for the removal of a brain tumor. She survived the operation but developed bronchial pneumonia and died on August 25, just a few weeks after my fifth birthday. She was thirty-eight.

Following my mother's death, some well-meaning soul told me since Mummy was such a good person, God needed her for an angel and had *taken* her to be with Him in heaven. I became angry at God for His selfishness in taking my mother from me. At five years of age, I came to the decision He was not to be trusted—*ever*.

For the next few weeks I spent many hours staring out of my bedroom window anxiously searching the skies—hoping I would be able to see my mother's soul on its way up to heaven. All I saw were birds flying, so I pretended she was a bird soaring up to heaven through the clouds and beyond.

In September 1950, at the age of five, I started school. Two weeks later, I came home sick with the measles. After that it was chickenpox, followed closely by numerous coughs and colds. The following January, I became seriously ill with whooping cough. My body burned with fever and I was weak from the constant coughing. The day came when the doctor told my family that if the fever didn't break, I would die within a few hours. I can still picture family members standing around my bed. I believe someone, somewhere must have prayed for me, because my fever broke that night and I recovered.

According to my sister, I was a sickly little kid, with stick-thin legs, sunken cheeks and tired-looking *racoon* eyes. She says it's a miracle I survived my early childhood.

~

I do remember *some* happy, carefree days spent building sand castles at the beach or playing with friends in our back yard. Without television, we enjoyed listening to children's stories on the radio. We created our own fun, playing with simple toys such as marbles and jacks. I had a pink-handled skipping rope and a favourite smooth, flat rock for playing hopscotch. My friends and I also passed many fun-filled hours playing beside the banks of the River Stour, throwing sticks and rocks into the water or catching minnows, frogs and tadpoles to take home in jam jars.

I have a wonderful memory of my brother taking me for a pony ride along River Way—not far from Granny Johnson's house. Dappled sunshine warmed us as we walked beneath a canopy of tall trees. My brother held the reigns firmly as he led the horse along the quiet street. I sat up straight in the saddle and held my head high, pretending I was Princess Elizabeth parading around Buckingham Palace. I have no memory of actually getting on or off this gentle brown horse, but the ride down River Way I'll never forget. To this day I still love horses.

Once I had recovered somewhat from all those early childhood illnesses I started to enjoy going to school. At the start of every school day, students lined up in the halls and paraded silently into the gym for morning assembly. Our teachers took turns reading from the Bible and organizing hymn singing and prayers. My favorite hymns were *All Things Bright and Beautiful* and *Onward Christian Soldiers.* Religious instruction was an important part of the school curriculum in those days. I especially loved the Bible stories about David and Goliath and Noah's ark.

Today I am appreciative of my early exposure to the basic history of Christianity. I believe God overlooked my childish resentment toward Him and allowed the Bible verses and words of those old hymns to stay with me and form the rock upon which my life would be built.

I thank you Lord, for keeping me
within the cleft of the rock.
My eyes were blind, I could not see,
but You knew what lay ahead for me.
When trouble came from all around,
You kept my feet on solid ground.

I also believe God honored my early baptism and protected my life. Even though I drifted far away from His presence, and literally became a lost soul, I somehow *knew* He was always there, patiently waiting for that day in the future when I would put aside my anger and hostility to walk willingly by His side.

~

A Temporary New Mother

For two years, Dad, with the help of my sixteen-year-old brother and twelve-year-old sister, attempted to keep the family together. In addition to his full-time job as an electrician, my father worked hard doing odd jobs for people in the neighbourhood. Whenever he worked for the local grocery store owner, he was paid in produce such as butter or bacon. I remember eating a lot of toast and *dripping* (fat left over after cooking bacon or the occasional Sunday roast). I also have a vivid memory of various food restrictions. Dad often reminded me, “Bread and jam or bread and butter, that’s all you can have.” To this day, I delight in having bread, butter *and* jam!

I knew we didn’t have much money. I hardly ever had any new clothes—however, I *was* fortunate enough to have two older cousins who provided me with numerous hand-me-down dresses and coats.

Most of the families on our quiet, tree-lined street cultivated large vegetable gardens and kept a few chickens to help make ends meet. I particularly enjoyed helping our neighbour, Mrs. Harris, prepare the feed for her chickens by mixing boiled potato peelings with some sort of bran. I loved squishing the mixture together in my hands until it was blended. Mrs. Harris would then walk with me to the chicken run, where I was allowed to feed the bran mixture to the chickens and collect the eggs. I felt very important to be trusted with this simple chore.

Dad eventually remarried. However, when his new wife became pregnant she either couldn't or wouldn't look after us. This resulted in my brother, sister and I being separated. Pat recently told me that, at age fourteen she actually ran away to live with our paternal grandmother. When Dad arrived to take my sister home with him, Granny locked her doors and sent him away empty-handed. My brother David, who was working as an apprentice heating and ventilating engineer, also left home at this time and found room and board with another family.

I was seven when Dad sent me to live with my Auntie Bee in West Drayton, Middlesex, on the outskirts of Greater London. He came home from work one day and asked me, "Who would you like to go stay with, Auntie Bee or Auntie Dorothy?" I liked Auntie Dorothy and my two cousins, but I was a bit scared of my Uncle Leslie, so I reluctantly chose Auntie Bee. I remember telling Dad, "I don't want to go away, I want to stay with you." I cried for hours and begged him not to send me away. He promised it would only be for a few weeks. Somehow, I didn't believe him. For the second time in my young life I made the decision not to trust, only this time it was my *earthly* father.

I soon discovered living with Auntie Bee was not so bad. She was a very kind person and I grew to love her dearly. Although she had never married, she loved children and would have made a great teacher. *(I always thought she had been jilted by a sailor, and I never dared to ask her why she had remained single. However, David recently told me that the sailor Auntie Bee loved was killed in the war.)* She did her best to give me every opportunity she could afford, including trips to London by train to see various musical productions and many visits to our favourite restaurant near Windsor Castle. We once saw the Queen and Princess Margaret drive by. I was also allowed to visit Lloyds Bank of London, where Auntie Bee worked.

It was Auntie Bee who taught me how to act in fine restaurants, which fork to pick up first, what to do with the napkin, how to eat soup correctly, etc. She also taught me how to make beds properly—with hospital corners. After Christmas and birthdays, she encouraged me to write thank-you letters for gifts received. Whenever I didn't know what to write, she would say, "Just write the first word—everything else will follow." I still do that today.

During the time we lived together, Auntie Bee became a Girl Guide Captain and I, rather reluctantly, joined the Girl Guides. Over the next four years, we enjoyed numerous camping trips and outings together and I met my very first best friend, Rosemary Hall. During the evenings Auntie Bee spent a great deal of time helping me with my math homework and on weekends she taught me how to plant flowers and grow vegetables. She also tried very hard to teach me about the love of God, but I wasn't ready to listen.

Auntie Bee (like my mother) was an excellent swimmer, and her determination that I learn to swim almost got me killed! One day I was standing at the edge of our local swimming pool watching other kids swimming, when someone accidently pushed me into the deep end. I stayed under for a long time. It was very blue down there and every time I opened my mouth, it seemed like I swallowed half the pool. Someone eventually fished me out and I survived the ordeal. Swimming lessons, with Auntie Bee close by my side, were a top priority after that. I did eventually learn how to swim. However where she swam *miles*, I only ever managed to swim *widths* of the pool. For the rest of my life, I never ventured anywhere near the deep end.

One thing I did enjoy was hearing about my mother's swimming accomplishments. Auntie Bee was happy to relate these stories to me. She told me growing up so close to the ocean was a lot of fun, and all three sisters became very strong swimmers. My favourite story has always been the one about my parents having a race. According to Auntie Bee, my mother used to swim from Boscombe Pier to Bournemouth Pier (a distance of approximately one-and-a-half miles) while my dad walked along the promenade. It didn't matter how fast my dad walked, Mummy always got to Bournemouth Pier ahead of him.

~

Auntie Bee did her best for me. Heaven knows I must have been a difficult child to raise. My rebellious outbursts tested her infinite patience many times. She worried about me when I wandered off to visit school friends without telling anyone where I was going. Auntie Bee's faith in God must have given her the strength to look after me. Even though she made sure I regularly said my prayers and attended church services, I was still not ready to forgive God for taking my mother to heaven. Anger and rebellion were always with me.

I didn't like the school in West Drayton so on sunny days I used to go sit in the park instead. Today, I would probably be labelled a juvenile delinquent. Back then, I was just a *troubled kid.* The other children sometimes teased me because of my skinny legs, but most of the time they just left me alone. One day at recess, a girl with long red hair started calling me names and tried to push me over. I grabbed her by the hair and threw her violently to the ground. No one messed with me after that!

When I was twelve, Auntie Bee became ill and Dad asked my brother and sister-in-law if they would look after me. They agreed and arrangements were made for me to return to Bournemouth once again. David was twenty-three years old at the time and had been married to Margaret for three years. They had a son Paul, who was two when I came to live with them. Their large, brick house was located in the village of Kinson, on the outskirts of Bournemouth. I was very happy to have a home with David and Margaret, and was determined to be better behaved. Once again, I started a new school and gradually settled down. School uniform was mandatory at Oakmead Girls School. I looked very smart in my white shirt, navy and green tie, navy skirt and white socks.

I enjoyed helping Margaret look after Paul. I took him for walks to the park and kept him amused. For much of his early childhood he was a very picky eater so we used all sorts of tricks and games to get him to eat his food.

Shortly after I moved back to Bournemouth, Auntie Bee visited us for a few days. I remember she slept in the single bed next to mine, and we talked late into the night, just like a couple of chatty school girls. At the time, I didn't know she was seriously ill. Later that year Auntie Bee was hospitalized and it was discovered she had inoperable stomach cancer. She died a few weeks later, at the age of forty-five.

When Auntie Bee died, I think part of me became numb. I don't remember feeling any kind of emotion. At the time it just seemed like everyone I loved either died or left me.

I have one of Auntie Bee's books in my bookcase, titled *When Man Listens* by Cecil Rose. The book is a description of the simple elements of Christian living and was first published in December 1936. Between the pages of this book, I found a small piece of paper with my aunt's handwritten commentary on Psalm 115. As a tribute to her memory, I have copied her exact words, as follows:

Psalm 115
Trust Thou in the Lord.

In those beautiful words the Psalmist sums up the secret of happiness, the folly of trusting and relying on material things and worldly gains and that the only way to live is to trust in the Lord. We have been reading about Daniel in our daily readings and surely he is a good example of one who absolutely trusted in God even when it meant what looked like a certain death. The secret of his absolute trust in God was the many times he spent quietly in prayer and communion with God. All down through the ages men and women have been guided and strengthened by those quiet times. That is how we can be guided and strengthened in the days to come.

[Written by Bertha Olive (Bee) Raines, prior to 1959]

The tears flowed as I typed these words and remembered her kindness to me, and for a few brief moments it seemed as if she was right beside me, bringing comfort one more time.

If I could say just a few words to her today they would be, *"I'm sorry for all the worry I caused you, and thank you for loving me."*

The Rescue

My niece Christine was born in August 1959. I remember rushing home from school every afternoon so I could take this adorable new baby for walks. I enjoyed showing her off to my friends. At that point in time, Christine became, in my eyes, the only human being who loved me as much as I loved her. It felt so safe to love a little child—after all, she was too young to die and leave me as Mummy and Auntie Bee had. As I helped take care of Christine, a loving bond developed between us. When she started walking, I was there holding my arms out to her. She learned to say my name at a very early age. I never minded getting into trouble for disciplining her older brother when he teased her. I was her protector. To this day, I'm convinced Christine validated my existence on this earth, and gave me a reason for living.

~

I have many fond memories of the seven years I lived with David and Margaret. We did everything as a family, whether it was a picnic, camping trip or vacation. On weekends we would visit nearby parks or go for walks along the beach. We often went for car rides in the country, but I was a very poor traveler and often became car sick. Many times on bus trips to Bournemouth, we would all have to get off long before our destination because I felt ill. My inability to travel well was a frustration for all concerned. At one time, my brother owned a rather old, very large Daimler car. It was like riding in a limousine (and for some reason it didn't make me sick).

At home, I constantly followed David around, eager to be his *helper*. In turn, he taught me how to paint, put up wallpaper, plant a garden and do all sorts of renovation jobs around the house. He also gave me my very first driving lesson at Holmesley Aerodrome where the old, unused runways provided the perfect place to practise.

In our garden we had a number of plum, pear and apple trees. Blackcurrent bushes also grew in abundance. I remember the batches of jam and jelly Margaret and I used to cook up. We also made fudge and peanut brittle. I can still visualize the small gas stove, the white enamel sink with wooden draining boards and the black tile floor of the old-style kitchen.

Life was relatively simple back then. Mothers stayed home to look after the children, clean house and cook meals. Dads went to work every day to earn money to keep the family supplied with food, clothing and shelter.

Margaret was very patient, teaching me everything young girls needed to learn in those days—like cooking, sewing and caring for children.

I enjoyed the role of auntie to Paul and Christine and my sister's two girls, Sally and Maryjane. I'll never forget the night Maryjane was born. Pat had asked me to sleep over because her husband Jack (a telephone operator) was working the night shift and if the baby came she needed someone to stay at home to look after two-year-old Sally.

At 1:30 in the morning, Pat nudged me and said, "I think the baby's coming." At fourteen, I knew nothing about delivering babies, so I quickly sent my sister off in an ambulance. Maryjane was born twenty minutes after Pat arrived at the maternity hospital!

Totally relieved that midwife duties hadn't been required of me, I went back to bed. Sally woke up early the next morning. After we ate breakfast I read stories to her until Jack came home from work.

I didn't think much about a career back then. It was just assumed I would one day marry and raise children.

When my nephew Stephen was born in December 1962, I was old enough to look after the household while Margaret was in the hospital. The piles of laundry were a bit daunting, but I managed OK. Needless to say, I was extremely happy to have her back home again at the end of the week.

I know I put David and Margaret through a lot of teenage turbulence in the early years, especially once I discovered boys. I also tried to smoke cigarettes but inhaling made me sick. They have since assured me I was no different from most other teenagers, including their own. They loved me and gave me a sense of stability. I'm still amazed when I consider their young age at the time they took me into their home.

When I was fourteen, I had the opportunity to take a two-year commercial course at school which included typing, shorthand, basic accounting and commerce. This meant an extra year for David and Margaret to support me (normally, school finished at age fifteen) but they agreed to it. In return, I put every effort into learning my lessons well. The fact that I excelled in shorthand and typing gave my self-esteem an incredible boost. When I completed the course at age sixteen, I was well prepared to begin my secretarial career and was soon hired by the accounting firm of Potter & Pollard as a junior typist. Earning wages for the first time in my life brought a great deal of satisfaction. I happily contributed part of my weekly wage to help out with the food bill, and delighted in being able to purchase my own clothes, such as high-heeled shoes with pointed toes, soft angora sweaters, and nylon stockings.

I didn't know it at the time but for the rest of my life,

earning a living became *the* most important source of personal security. Whenever the ability to earn money was threatened (through illness, pregnancy, etc.) I had a tendency to fall apart.

CHAPTER TWO

Friends and Neighbours

God sets the lonely in families,
he leads forth the prisoners with singing...
~Psalm 68:6

In the summer of 1961 a new family moved in next door to David and Margaret's house in Kinson. Our new neighbours, Lily and Stan, had decided to move to Bournemouth from Southampton shortly after their 25th wedding anniversary. Stan had a new job as manager of one of the elite men's clothing stores in Bournemouth. They had two teenagers around my age. Their son, John was older, already married and living in Southampton. I liked Lily and Stan right away and soon became friends with their daughter Jennifer. It turned out she would also be attending Oakmead Girls School, so we walked to school together. It was wonderful having Jennifer for a friend. She was smart and beautiful. She had this amazing red hair (which all the boys raved over) and if that wasn't enough, her brother Martin was really good-looking. Jennifer and I spent a lot of time together before we started dating boys. They were fun times.

One day when I came home from school, Martin was in

their front yard tinkering with his motorbike. He started chatting to me over the fence. "Do you like Ella Fitzgerald?" he asked me.

"Oh yes, she's great," I replied, and ran indoors blushing crimson!

"Margaret, who's Ella Fitzgerald?" I blurted out the moment I saw her in the kitchen.

"She's a singer with an amazing voice—why?"

"Martin just asked me."

"Martin?"

"The boy next door."

"Oh!"

As luck would have it, she was too busy in the kitchen to notice my blushing cheeks, or I would have been teased! I ran upstairs and flopped down on my bed to daydream about this handsome neighbour.

After that, I spent a great deal of time next door talking with Jennifer, Martin and his parents. They had this wonderful air of stability and kindness about them. I couldn't quite put my finger on it, but it drew me into their home time and time again. To me they were a whole, normal family who cared about each other. I desperately wanted what they had.

Of course, I loved my home with David and Margaret and the children. However when you're a teenager, home usually means homework, chores and responsibilities. At Martin's house I was free of all that and could just have fun. It didn't take long for me to embrace his whole family with a deep and lasting affection.

Martin and I dated for three weeks that summer. However, it would be more than two years before we went out together again. It was actually Martin's mom who played cupid. As it happened, Martin needed a date for a

Christmas dance. His mom suggested he ask me to go with him. To cut a long story short, his mom talked to Margaret, Margaret talked to me, and I agreed to go to the dance with him. I wore Margaret's pale blue chiffon dress, cinched in at the waist by a dark blue sash. I spent most of the evening trying to prevent the dress from slipping off my narrow shoulders. However, this didn't stop Martin and I from having a great time together. We both enjoyed good music and loved to dance.

From that night on, we began dating seriously. Martin took me everywhere on the back of his motorbike, and I loved it. When I look back now at the crazy stunts we pulled on that bike, it's a miracle we lived through it. One time we leaned over so far in a turn, sparks flew as the kick-stand scraped the edge of the curb. Then there was the time the headlamp quit working. We were driving along a country road late at night and had to slow to a crawl in an attempt to see where we were going. One time we overtook a bus when another bus was coming toward us. We squeaked through the gap with a couple of inches to spare.

We were young, in love, and absolutely mad!

Martin and I were married at St. Andrew's Church in Kinson, two months prior to my 20th birthday. With Margaret's help, I sewed my own wedding dress and the dresses for our four little nieces who were bridesmaids. Martin printed the invitations at his work. Following a simple brunch reception at the Wincroft Hotel at Ferndown, we honeymooned for a week at the Bancourt Hotel in Torquay, Devon. On our arrival, we discovered our bedroom was right above the kitchen. All we could hear was the constant clatter of dishes! The first morning of our honeymoon was spent removing all the *Just Married* stickers Martin's work-mates had pasted all over our car, which I believe, was a 1946 Austin. I do know it was ancient and extremely unreliable. It often stalled going up steep hills and if we did manage to make it up the hill, there was always a distinct possibility the brakes would overheat going down the other side.

Our first home together was three furnished rooms in the upper level of a house in Winton near Bournemouth. The place was very old and drafty. We had to share the bathroom with the landlord and his wife. I remember we were only allowed to have one bath a week each—to conserve the hot water, I guess. Sometimes we would trick the landlord by having a bath together, so that we could have *two* baths a week each! We also had to put shilling coins in a gas meter to use the gas stove in the kitchen. During the winter months the place was freezing cold, so we used to huddle in the kitchen and turn on the gas stove to keep warm.

I don't think we cared much about *creature comforts* in those days. We were content just being together. Neither of us looked too far into the future. I was happy to be married and belong to someone. Martin was good to me. Occasionally, I would get angry or upset when my feelings were hurt by something he said or did. At these times, I would go for a long walk until I had calmed down. For the most part, I enjoyed our early days together tremendously.

Neither of us anticipated the life journey we were about to take would reveal the fragility of my emotions in the years to come.

CHAPTER THREE

Adventure, With a Price to Pay

Early in 1966, my brother started talking about emigrating to Canada. We all learned as much as we could about the country and its people. We were especially interested in the Canadian climate. When Martin and I read in various pamphlets about the low temperatures in winter, we actually thought they must be printing errors!

I don't know how David convinced Margaret to leave her home and family but he did. A few months later we were saying tearful goodbyes and wishing them well as they left England with their three children and much luggage, for a new life in Sarnia, Ontario, Canada.

Somewhere along the way, David had also convinced Martin and me of the benefits of a new life in Canada. The timing was perfect, as Martin was just about to complete a four-year printing apprenticeship. We started saving as much money as we could from my salary. Martin was enthusiastic about applying to emigrate to Canada. As a fully trained printer and secretary, with youth on our side and in excellent health, our application was readily accepted. To save the rent money we moved in with his parents for the last few weeks before leaving England. Martin managed to get a job as a type-setter with a farming magazine in Saskatoon, Saskatchewan, so that became our final destination.

Now it was our turn to say tearful goodbyes to our family. My sister Pat was heartbroken. In a few short weeks she had been parted from her brother and family, and now her sister and husband were leaving too. Saying goodbye to my sister, her husband and my two nieces was one of the hardest things I have ever done. As we drove away from their house, it was a very sad time for all of us.

On June 23, 1966, we boarded a plane at Heathrow Airport, bound for Canada. With brief stops in Montreal and Winnipeg, and a very bumpy flight from Winnipeg to Saskatoon (through a thunderstorm), we finally landed safely. We had arrived! Our only possessions were two suitcases crammed full of clothes, a trunk filled with wedding presents, $600 and a small birdcage containing our pet parakeet.

We spent our first few days in Saskatoon looking for a place to live. We settled on a sparsely furnished basement suite in the southeast section of the city. Martin started work right away and a few days later, I got a typing job with the Department of Human Resources. In the beginning we thought we would die of the heat, and then as summer progressed into winter, we thought we would freeze to death!

In a letter to David and Margaret, we promised to drive down to Sarnia for a weekend soon (not realizing it would take more than a weekend to actually drive there). However, as December drew near, we couldn't face spending our first Christmas in Canada without them, so Martin and

I decided we would drive to Sarnia for a week between Christmas and New Year's. We shared the driving with another couple who also had family close to Sarnia.

To say it was a long drive is the understatement of the century. We endured snow, ice, fatigue, faulty tires, halucinations, did I say fatigue? At one point, literally in the middle of nowhere, we pulled off the road, only to break through the snow and slide into the ditch. We didn't understand the complexities of snow grading—we thought there was firm ground at the edge of the road. Lucky for us a truck stopped and the driver very kindly pulled our car out of its snowy resting place with the use of chains. It was the first time in our lives we had watched a truck pull a car out of the ditch!

For the last fifty miles, the only way we could stay awake was to open all the windows and sing Christmas carols.

Finally we arrived. It was wonderful to see David, Margaret and the children. However, we were so tired, we went straight to bed and slept for ten hours. The week went by quickly. We enjoyed tobogganing and visiting local points of interest. The drive back to Saskatoon was grueling, but we got home safely.

The vastness of the land really hit home—this was a *really big* country!

~

The following Spring, Martin found out the newspaper in Rocky Mountain House, Alberta, was looking for an experienced printer. He applied for the job and received a reply almost immediately saying his application was successful. We gave notice to both our employers, packed everything we owned into our car and headed west.

Adventure, with a Price to Pay

We had never lived in a small town before. The people were very friendly and introduced us to that wonderful event called a potluck supper. Everyone, it seemed, had their own favourite recipe. I kept small scraps of paper in my purse in order to write them down. The ones that stand out in my mind are for meatballs, meatloaf and various types of dessert squares. I stayed away from the pork hocks! It was a very different life for us but we enjoyed it nevertheless. We found a nice suite in a fourplex and bought some furniture. I started work as a teller trainee at a local bank.

On the weekends we drove for miles on back-country gravel roads enjoying the vast open spaces. As we looked around us at the mountains, rivers, fields and farms, the sheer beauty of it all thrilled us. We felt invincible and confident. Surely success was within our grasp. The future looked good.

~

Toward the end of February 1967, I started feeling sick in the mornings and we realized I was pregnant. The sickness got worse. I couldn't even suck an ice-cube or brush my teeth without throwing up! I had to give up my teller job and was eventually hospitalized and fed intravenously for a few days in an effort to settle my stomach.

When I came home from the hospital, Martin presented me with a cute little black terrier puppy. We named her Tiny. She was so small that the only way she could eat was by putting her two front paws into the food dish.

A few weeks later, Martin heard about a better paying job at the newspaper in Red Deer, Alberta and thought it would be a good move for us. We packed up our belongings once more and loaded them into a rented trailer, which we towed with our car. In Red Deer we lived in a basement suite for a few weeks until we were able to purchase our first home (a three-bedroom rancher, which cost only $11,000).

Martin settled into his new job and we started making friends. I was now well into my fourth month of pregnancy and still battling the nausea. Gradually, my stomach settled down somewhat, but my body (and brain) had lacked nutrition for a long period of time. I started having nightmares that when our baby was born, it wouldn't be able to breathe. I gradually slipped into a severe depression.

Shortly after that, I started worrying about our finances. Even with the better paying job, money was in short supply. With only Martin working, I was concerned we wouldn't be able to provide the necessary clothes and crib for the coming baby. No one around me realized the depths of my anxiety.

One morning shortly after Martin had gone to work, I took an overdose of tranquilizers desiring only to end my suffering, fall asleep and never wake up. Thank heavens, Martin decided to come home at lunchtime that day and found me unconscious. I was rushed to the hospital by ambulance to have my stomach pumped. A hospital psychiatrist tried to get me to talk to him, but I was uncooperative. The next day I was discharged and Martin brought me home. After that, our neighbour checked on me once or twice a day while Martin was at work.

I had been home from the hospital for a few days when a social worker contacted me. She had heard about my illness and depression and managed to get me a temporary three-week job working for the Minister of the United Church, Reverend Oldring. I really enjoyed working for him for those three weeks. Now, at last, I had some money for baby clothes.

Martin and I started going to Sunday services at Gaetz United Church in Red Deer and attended membership classes led by Reverend Oldring. For reasons I do not understand, my depression lifted. I managed to endure the rest of my pregnancy without too much discomfort, although I still experienced the same nightmare occasionally.

For my birthday that year, Martin bought me a white leather bound King James Bible. I know he was at a loss to even begin to understand what I had gone through emotionally, but as he handed me the Bible, he said, "I hope this will help to give you strength." I thanked him without realizing the future importance of the gift. I had actually wanted him to buy me a maternity dress. The Bible was hardly touched over the next seventeen years. Today, however, its cover is worn from constant use, the edges starting to tear. Many pages are stained with oil from my fingers, where I have turned those particular pages so often. The Bible Martin gave me for my 22nd birthday is still the one I use the most. Placed on my bedside table at night and my coffee table during the day, it is always within close reach. In the event of a house fire—my King James Bible and the cat get rescued first!

~

Around three o'clock in the morning on November 17, 1967, I went into labor. After a difficult birth (when his heart-rate dropped to dangerously low levels) our baby boy had some problems with fluid in his lungs and stopped breathing many times. Each time, the doctors were able to revive him. Frantic that our baby might die without being baptized, I asked Martin to contact Reverend Oldring. He came to the hospital immediately and baptized the tiny baby we had named Carl. I can still picture the three of us standing around the incubator as little Carl struggled to breathe. The doctors did everything they could to keep reviving him, but on the third day of his short life, our baby died. Little Carl was born on November 17, lived through November 18, and died on November 19, 1967. Martin and I were heartbroken and numb with grief.

The nurses made a valiant attempt to move me to another ward, but there were no other beds available. That night, alone in my room, I could hear babies crying in the nursery down the hall. It was the longest night of my life. The next morning, I begged my doctor to discharge me and let me go home. He agreed.

In the meantime, Martin had the horrendous task of phoning relatives to inform them of Carl's death.

A few weeks after Carl's funeral, the representative from the funeral home came to our house to ask us what inscription we wanted carved onto the baby's headstone. Without hesitation, I uttered these words, *"Safe in the arms of Jesus."*

~

Two Precious Gifts from God

Reverend Oldring was a great comfort to us in the months following Carl's death and we continued to attend Sunday services at the United Church regularly. Struggling with grief and an immense sense of loss, I appreciated the kind-ness and outreach of church women as they telephoned or stopped in to visit me.

I wanted to return to work as soon as possible and started checking the *help wanted* section of the newspaper. I managed to get a secretarial job with a local life insurance company. Slowly, day-by-day, our lives resumed without little Carl.

Adventure, with a Price to Pay

In 1969 we sponsored Martin's parents so they could come to Canada. I was very happy to have them with us. Martin's dad got a job at a local men's clothing store and his mum started working part-time at the Red Deer library. They rented an apartment a couple of blocks from us and adapted easily to their new life in Canada.

That summer, Martin and I started talking about adopting a baby. We were both employed, owned our home and loved children. Martin said, "We are two people who need a child. Surely there will be a child somewhere who needs *us*." He was right! We started the application process in September, enduring interviews, home visits and health checks on both of us. We had no spectacular demands. We just asked for *a baby*! The weeks of waiting seemed to drag by slowly. Then, just two days before Christmas 1969, we were notified a baby boy was available for us in Edmonton. The next day dawned cold and frosty, but with a bright blue Alberta sky. We drove up to Edmonton with great excitement and brought home our new son, Elliot. When we found out his date of birth, we just knew he was meant to be ours. He was born on November 18, 1969, which was the only complete day our little Carl had lived two years earlier.

I was fortunate to have Martin's mum close by to help me in those early days of motherhood, because Elliot was a fussy baby. Even after bathing, feeding, burping and changing his diaper, he would always scream for ten minutes before he'd fall asleep! I'm sure he must have suffered some kind of emotional trauma being separated from his birth mother. Many nights we used to take him for car rides so the motion would lull him to sleep. When we took Elliot for walks, people stopped to admire his olive skin, dark brown eyes and wavy black hair. We were very proud parents!

At last we felt like a proper family. I was particularly content. I had my in-laws close by. David and Margaret were now living in Edmonton, and we could visit them often. I had a comfortable home. Martin was also doing gardening work for people on the weekends to earn extra money.

Even though I took a break from full-time work for the next seven years, I never again experienced the anxiety I had endured when I was pregnant with Carl.

In February 1970, I started feeling sick in the mornings and thought I had the 'flu. I went to see Dr. Craigie and he laughingly told me to go home and start knitting baby booties. Yes, I was pregnant! Before I left his office, however, I persuaded him to give me a prescription for medication to stop the nausea. Thankfully, this pregnancy was much easier than the first. Of course, I fully realized Elliot and the new baby would be close in age but I felt confident everything would turn out fine. Now that I had family close by, I could relax.

In the summer of 1970, David and Margaret sold their house in Edmonton and moved to Kamloops, B.C. I missed our regular visits and partially consoled myself with the knowledge that Kamloops was much closer than Sarnia.

~

As the months passed, I happily immersed myself in domesticity and motherhood. However, unknown to me, Martin had his hopes set on purchasing a small weekly newspaper and printing business in Didsbury, Alberta (a farming community about an hour's drive south of Red Deer). When he finally told me about it, I was not happy with the idea at all. I definitely had no desire to leave my home or Martin's parents in Red Deer. *What did he think he was doing?* We had a six-month-old baby, with another on the way. I dug my heels in and refused to move. In the heated arguments that followed, I was adamant. I would not move again. The thought of giving up the security of a regular paycheque was unnerving, to say the least. Martin, on the other hand, was eager to be his own boss. He promised to find us a decent place to live. He assured me we could visit his parents every weekend if I wanted. Determined to win me over to his way of thinking, he promised the world.

We finally settled for a new mobile home in the middle of a field on the southeast corner of Didsbury. However, I was *not* a happy camper! Once again I found myself living in a new location, with few friends and many responsibilities. On the bright side, Elliot brought great comfort to me as I watched him grow into a strong, healthy toddler.

Our lovely little house in Red Deer sold quickly and, for better or worse, we became the owners of a printing business.

At this point in our lives, Martin may have won the battle over where we lived, but he lost the war. Resentment toward him started to build in my heart. Life was never the same again. Gradually, I began to shut him out and concentrated my attentions on our son.

In October 1970, my doctor sent me to Calgary Foothills Hospital to await the imminent birth. He wanted to ensure nothing went wrong. I actually loved being in the hospital. I enjoyed talking with the other women in my room. It was an oasis of sorts—a place where I had no worries or concerns. All I had to do was relax and before too long, give birth to the enormous bulge in my stomach! The morning of October 16, I started to go into labour and was transferred to the delivery ward. The nurse asked me if I wanted her to telephone my husband. I told her not to bother. I knew it was a Thursday morning and he would be driving up to Red Deer to get the newspaper printed.

After just a few hours of mild cramps, and one humongous pain, I gave birth to a beautiful healthy baby girl.

As the nurse was cleaning me up after the delivery, she asked me if I would like anything to eat or drink.

"I'd love some tea and toast, with butter *and* jam please," I replied. A few minutes later, she came back with everything I had asked for. That was the best tea and toast I had ever tasted in my life!

Then she asked me an odd question. She said, "Are you ready?"

I asked her, "Ready for what?"

She then explained, "Your specialist likes his patients to *walk* back to their ward after they've given birth."

I thought she was joking, but she had this *no nonsense* look in her eye! Helping me down from the bed, she followed close behind with a wheelchair (just in case) as I proceeded to *walk* unaided down the long corridor which led to my ward. When I entered my room, the other women couldn't believe I had just given birth to a baby girl. Our ward nurse came in at that moment and confirmed my story. As she helped me get into bed, she whispered to me, "I'd like to see *him* (referring to my specialist) give birth to a seven-pound baby and *walk* back to *his* room afterwards!" When I told the other women what she had said, we all collapsed into fits of uncontrollable laughter.

I could have stayed in the hospital with those women for ever. I certainly wasn't anxious to go home. Home meant meals, laundry, two babies, a workaholic husband and little chance of fellowship with anyone. However, the day soon came when Martin arrived to take us home and I had to say goodbye to my new friends.

We named our baby girl Michaela Joy. Unlike her slightly older brother, she was a peaceful baby and slept through the night at a very early age. It didn't take long for us to notice the personality differences in our children. Elliot was definitely an adventuresome mischief-maker while Michaela was a quiet, contented child.

Our living arrangements were cramped to say the least. If it wasn't for my kind neighbor, Shirley, I probably would have gone quite mad. She helped me greatly by allowing me to visit her *large* farmhouse frequently for coffee, and listened patiently as I poured out my frustrations.

Martin's parents drove down to Didsbury most weekends and we enjoyed their company tremendously. They both adored their grandchildren. Many times, Martin's dad would phone me and say, "I'll drive down, if you make roast beef and Yorkshire pudding for supper." I always did.

We often stayed up late playing cards. I seemed to be the first person to get tired and want to quit. One night, when I went into the kitchen to make tea, Martin turned the living room clock back an hour to trick me into playing cards longer. It worked!

For the next few months Martin devoted his time and energy to the printing business, while I concentrated on looking after our two young children. The mobile home was no longer a suitable place for two toddlers, so we sold it and bought an older home in Carstairs, ten miles south of Didsbury. It was good to have a proper garden again and more living space. Through a series of events, Martin decided to sell the Didsbury operation to the man who owned the other Didsbury newspaper. We took over the printing of the Carstairs News. Over the next six years we developed it into a successful printing and weekly newspaper business.

It was at the print shop in Carstairs that Martin taught me how to cut and paste, display advertising, operate many different types of printing and typesetting equipment and set type for newspapers and books. As well as running the business, Martin also drove a school bus, served a term on the town council and was a volunteer fireman.

Our friends, Marge and Clarence owned the local variety store. They were a great help to us during our years in Carstairs. Clarence also drove a school bus and served on the town council. I remember Marge always used to help me by keeping Elliot and Michaela amused while I spent a few minutes wandering around the store.

It was also in Carstairs that our children played happily and in safety on local streets and playgrounds. Everyone watched out for their neighbors. I never had to worry about locking my door. It was a safe, friendly place to live.

In 1976 Martin started a printing business in Calgary and sold the Carstairs News. We rented a large, modern house located in the north-west section of Calgary. This would be our last home together. When Martin's Dad died suddenly of a heart attack in June 1977, we had no reason to keep up the illusion of a happily married couple. We separated a month later.

It's difficult to explain now—a quarter of a century later—how Martin and I grew apart. Somehow, we became two separate and totally different human beings who really didn't like each other very much.

I will always wonder if our separation and eventual divorce could have been avoided if we had learned to apply just one Biblical teaching to our marriage. I'm particularly thinking of the excellent advice contained in Ephesians,

Adventure, with a Price to Pay

chapter four:

Get rid of all bitterness, rage and anger... Be kind and compassionate to one another, forgiving each other, just as in Christ, God forgave you.

~

Four Minus Two

In July 1977, I left Calgary with two children, four suitcases and two large boxes of toys. The kind woman who checked our luggage at Calgary Airport didn't charge me one cent for overweight baggage. As the plane taxied for takeoff en route to Vancouver, B.C., Elliot leaned over me and told his sister in a very loud voice, "You'd better hold mom's hand, you know she hates takeoffs." Everyone within hearing distance cracked up laughing—while I turned a bright shade of red!

Martin's brother John, wife Eileen and three daughters had emigrated to British Columbia in 1967. Now they kindly offered a temporary refuge for Elliot, Michaela and myself in their spacious North Vancouver home. Eileen met me at Vancouver Airport and helped me load two rather unsettled children and mounds of luggage into her car.

Within a few days of our arrival in Vancouver, I managed to get a full-time secretarial job with a local bank. Eileen spent most of that summer at the beach with her three girls, as well as Elliot and Michaela. Both John and Eileen were very kind to us through this emotional time and certainly were a great help to me as I struggled to get my life in order.

Three weeks later, Martin drove out to Vancouver with some of our furniture and personal effects. He also decided to live in North Vancouver. As the school year approached,

Martin began asking me if he could have custody of Elliot. I wasn't sure what to do. I loved both my children desperately, but was filled with fear. I didn't know if I was strong enough to survive with one child, let alone two. I was very much afraid of what the future held for me. Certainly in those days, I had little faith, and therefore, little hope.

In the end Elliot went to live with his dad and I made sure he spent every other weekend with us.

Michaela and I moved to Surrey and ended up living in the same apartment building as my niece Christine and her husband Stephen. Christine was studying to be a lab technologist at the British Columbia Institute of Technology. It was comforting once more to have family close by, especially when David and Margaret came to visit. When Michaela started grade one, she met her best friend Liz. I became good friends with Liz's mom, Roanne. Elliot spent every other weekend with us and I cried many tears on Sunday nights when he returned to his Dad's place.

In February 1978, I started work at a bank in Coquitlam. Shortly after that, Michaela and I moved to an apartment close to my work. The next few years were spent working hard and struggling to make ends meet financially. My net pay was around $750 per month and my apartment rent was $300. Groceries, car expenses and clothing costs took care of the rest. I bought some used furniture from one of my co-workers who allowed me to pay her back at $50 per month. On pay days (every other Friday) Michaela and I usually went to McDonald's for supper. At other times, when money was short, we ate Kraft Dinner, spaghetti, or sausages and baked beans. I quickly figured out—if I wrote a cheque for groceries on a Wednesday night, it didn't clear my bank account until *after* my pay was deposited. To this day, I have no idea how Michaela and I survived, but somehow we made it through.

Everyone in the family knew to send us clothes for birthday presents!

In the years that followed, John and Eileen continued to keep in close contact with us, providing a strong sense of family togetherness. Their many acts of kindness and generosity played a large part in helping me approach life with increased self-confidence.

Thankfully, my job was stable in those days (prior to downsizing). Over the years I advanced to Senior Steno, then Senior Word Processor. With regular pay increases, life for Michaela and I became a little easier. In the last six years of my career I provided secretarial support to the Community Banking Manager. This position of trust and responsibility gave me the financial security I had always desired.

When David and Margaret moved to Victoria in September 1978, Elliot, Michaela and I visited them often. Their home was always a safe haven for us—a place where we could be with family and have fun.

CHAPTER FOUR

Turning Around

Come to me, all you who are weary and burdened, and I will give you rest. Take my yoke upon you and learn from me, for I am gentle and humble in heart, and you will find rest for your souls. For my yoke is easy and my burden is light.
~Matthew 11:28-30

For most of my life I had been angry at God—having decided at a very early age He was not to be trusted. I had gone my own way and only grudgingly acknowledged Him over the years with small *tokens* of respect by getting married in church and making sure my children were baptized.

In a continuous search for something or someone to *make me happy,* I joined a single parents group and went to meetings and dances. I became selfish and self-absorbed. I dated selfish and self-absorbed men. I drank some and partied a lot. I also read self-help books and attended all kinds of seminars on inner healing and assertiveness training. However, I always ended up coming face to face with my own inadequacies and shortcomings. My life had no real purpose and I could find no solution to improving my empty existence. When I finally came to the end of *self,* I was divorced, angry, rebellious and thirty-eight years old!

It wasn't until I met Kaye that I learned the truth of God's amazing love and forgiveness.

Working as a bank receptionist, I met all kinds of people. Kaye, however, stood out from the crowd. She always had a smile on her face. Her whole countenance seemed to glow. The only annoying trait about her was that she loved to talk about church. Whenever I tried to tell her about my latest trip down the road of self-help, she would somehow turn the conversation around to the previous Sunday's sermon. To this day, I don't know how she did it. We laugh about it now, but at the time I remember getting quite angry and upset with her. Of course, she'd always forgive me and I couldn't stay mad at her for long.

Back in 1984, I had no idea this amazing woman and her family would come to mean so much to me or that God had a special plan for both of us.

Jesus was gently knocking on the door of my heart and waiting patiently for me to let Him in.

In the meantime, unknown to the relatives living in Canada, my sister in England had become a Christian and boldly asked the ladies in her newly-formed Bible study group to pray for my salvation! Thanks to the dedication of those dear women, the power of prayer from halfway around the world was about to change my life forever.

At the time I was entangled in yet another unsatisfactory relationship. When I experienced the call of God, it felt like having someone catch hold of me and point out, in no uncertain terms, my life was headed in the wrong direction. What actually happened was I simply got out of bed one Sunday morning and told my boyfriend I just had to go to church!

He looked up at me sleepily and mumbled, "Church? Are

you crazy? What's got into you all of a sudden?"

In all honesty, I said, "I don't know what's got into me. I just feel like going to church." Not wishing to get into an argument, I hastily grabbed my clothes and purse and headed for the bathroom, adding firmly, "I am *going* to church." With that, I showered, dressed, grabbed a muffin from the kitchen counter and literally *ran* out the front door.

Needless to say, the relationship didn't last very long after that!

When I drove away from the house that Sunday morning, I had no idea where to go. Then I remembered reading in one of the local newspapers that Reverend Oldring was now the minister of a church in New Westminster. I drove around the unfamiliar streets until I saw his name on a billboard outside a church building. I parked my car, took a deep breath and walked down the path to the main entrance of the church. Reverend Oldring and his wife Joy were happy to see me again after so many years. Naturally, they asked me about Martin and were saddened to hear of our divorce.

I sat through the service, drinking in every word. After the final hymn everyone held hands to sing "I'll pray for you, if you pray for me, until we meet again." This simple chorus made me cry. (It's impossible to wipe the tears from your eyes when you have someone on either side of you holding your hand!)

I attended Reverend Oldring's church regularly. His sermons ministered to my wounded spirit and each Sunday I learned more about God. As the weeks passed, I knew I would have to tell Kaye what I had been doing.

Early one Monday morning, she phoned me at work.

"How would you like to go out for lunch today?"

"I'd love to." I replied eagerly—I had so many questions to ask her.

For the next three hours, the rain poured and the wind blew. I was sure Kaye would cancel, but no, she arrived promptly at noon carrying a very large, sturdy umbrella. We walked up the street to the restaurant together. When we sat down at our table, I couldn't help but blurt out, "Kaye, I've been going to church for quite a few weeks now, but at the end of the service, I still feel hungry for something more." She looked at me and smiled knowingly. "That *something more* is a person" she said gently. "His name is JESUS."

"You'd better come to church with me on Saturday," she added. "There's an evangelist coming to speak. My husband and I will take you." I wondered if I was ready to listen to an evangelist, but Kaye's enthusiasm must have rubbed off on me because I said "Yes." I knew in my heart I trusted Kaye completely and I desperately wanted the joy and peace that she had found in her relationship with God.

She blessed the food set before us, grinned at me and said, "Now, eat your pizza."

As promised, Kaye and her husband Earl picked me up on the Saturday evening and drove me to the meeting. As we entered the school auditorium, I looked around in amazement. I had never seen so many joyous, smiling people in one place before. The meeting began with singing followed by prayer. Then the evangelist gave his message. To this day, I can't remember what he spoke about. However, when he invited people to come forward if they wanted to receive more from Jesus, I knew he was talking to me!

Kaye's eyes were wet with tears of joy when I left my seat and walked to the front of the auditorium. I wasn't alone. There were at least twenty other searching souls up there with me. A lady came and stood behind me and we were ushered into a large room behind the stage. We sat at a small table. She read some verses from her Bible and talked to me for a while. Then she asked me if I would like to ask Jesus to forgive me of my sins! Well, I knew in my heart I wasn't living right, but for one long minute I hesitated and a voice in my brain seemed to be telling me *"Pauline, you're not that bad."* Finally, I said *"YES. I want to ask Jesus to forgive me of my sins."* When I spoke the words out loud, I felt a warmth flow through my body from the top of my head to the soles of my feet.

A gentle feeling of peace seemed to wash over me. I realized what a tiresome strain it had been to keep pushing God away. Now I knew beyond a shadow of a doubt I had been forgiven, cleansed and set free. My thirty-eight years of *wilderness experiences* were ended.

I had become a child of God!

~

The next morning I woke up early and decided to tidy up the flower bed outside my apartment. Over the winter many weeds had grown in the large raised box of earth I shared with the apartment next door. I got out a trowel, gardening gloves and large plastic bag and went to work. It was a beautiful, sunny April day. I hummed some of the choruses I had heard the night before. My task completed, I brought in the trowel and gloves and was about to close the patio door when an inner voice seemed to whisper, "Why have you only pulled the weeds from *your* side of the flower bed and haven't touched your neighbour's side?" I nervously turned and glanced over my shoulder, half expecting to *actually see* someone, but I was alone.

Turning Around

I knew I didn't want to be seen clambering onto my neighbour's patio early on a Sunday morning, but I also knew this was *day one* of being a Christian, so I grabbed the trowel and gloves, took a quick peak outside to make sure no one was around and proceeded to weed my neighbour's half of the flower bed. I came back inside and realized it was time to shower and get ready for church. A few minutes later, in the middle of showering, my mind was flooded with words and melody, so precious and beautiful, I jumped out of the shower, grabbed a towel and ran to my kitchen table (dripping water all the way). With great excitement, I hastily wrote down this, my very first message of comfort and inspiration from God:

God is good, so good, praise Him, praise Him.
For His light shines through, for me and you.
God is good, so good, praise Him evermore!

God is love, pure love, praise Him, praise Him.
For His light shines through, for me and you,
God is love, pure love, praise Him evermore!

God brings peace to all, praise Him, praise Him.
For His light shines through, for me and you,
God brings peace to all, praise Him evermore!

A simple act of obedience to a gently whispered instruction brought me a blessing that not only helped me to realize God is real, but that He loves me! This previously hopeless *woman at the well* had found the truth, and was set free to worship and praise the One who had waited so patiently and lovingly for her.

For the next few months (much to the consternation of

my family and *some* of my friends) all I did was read my Bible and listen to Christian radio programs. I had some good talks with Reverend Oldring and he understood completely when I told him I wanted to attend church with my friends. He certainly played an important role in preparing my heart to receive the message spoken by the evangelist—proving the truth of 1 Corinthians 3:7 & 8:

> *So neither he who plants nor he who waters is anything, but only God, who makes things grow. The man who plants and the man who waters have one purpose, and each will be rewarded according to his own labour.*

Kaye and Earl nurtured me through the next few months. They answered all my questions and guided me always with the truth of God's word. As a fledgling Christian, I made many mistakes but Kaye and Earl always brought me back to the cross and what Jesus had accomplished for us there. I realized I had been holding onto some of my old, worldly ways and this was preventing true growth as a Christian. One day I knelt on my living room floor and had a *heart-to-heart* talk with the Lord. I knew a crossroads had been reached and the right path must be chosen. I told the Lord, "I don't want anything the world has to offer, I just want to follow you." Life was much easier after that.

I read my King James Bible at every opportunity. The words were alive with promise, healing, hope and love. I gradually found answers to every life question within its pages.

As I grew in my Christian walk, I began to understand that Jesus had experienced more pain and suffering than I had. A whole new respect and reverence for Him began to grow in my heart.

I stopped being angry at God. The word FATHER took on a whole new meaning. Reading about Christ's death on the cross, I came to the realization my heavenly Father and I had something in common. I had watched my infant son die, He had watched His adult son die. We had a bond for eternity.

As I pursued a deeper relationship with the Lord, words of adoration and praise for my Saviour poured out of my bruised and battered heart, filling whatever scraps of paper I could find to write on.

The poem Spiritual Awakening is one of my earliest writings:

I used to be a troubled soul,
wrapped up in a cocoon
of doubt and insecurity,
I never really saw the moon
or stars so bright
or enjoyed a sunny day,
I was trapped by many problems
that wouldn't go away.

Then came a light
so strong and bright
the anxiousness of old
retreated from my trembling heart
and I became quite bold.

Removing the Sting

All fear and doubt
just slipped away
like mist on a sunny morn.
I'm glad the light
shone bright for me
and I could be reborn.

CHAPTER FIVE

Friends Together

My command is this: Love each other as I have loved you. Greater love has no one than this, that he lay down his life for his friends. You are my friends if you do what I command.
~John 15:12-14

In the Fall of 1984, I heard about a Christian singles conference to be held at Broadway Pentecostal Tabernacle in Vancouver. I was curious. When someone at Kaye's church gave me the information brochure, I decided to complete the registration form and send it in.

Arriving a few minutes early on the day of the conference, I slipped into the washroom to freshen up. As I combed my hair and checked myself over in the mirror, I noticed a fair-haired woman beside me doing the very same thing. I think we were both hoping to meet Mr. tall, dark, handsome and Christian. I smiled at her and we started talking about the conference. We agreed to sit together, and ended up listening to the same speakers for much of the day. The woman's name was Donna and she had been a Christian for three weeks. I had by that time been a Christian for just about six months *(so, of course, I knew everything!)*

In spite of my *overbearing zeal,* this chance meeting in a church washroom blossomed into a friendship which has remained strong to this day. Donna and I joined the Broadway singles group and attended church there. We were both baptized on February 17, 1985, and grew up in faith together.

Also, in July 1985, my son Elliot came back to live with us. He was eager to complete grades eleven and twelve at Centennial High School in Coquitlam. I was just happy to have him in our lives again on a full-time, permanent basis. I thanked God for this second chance with my son and promised—with His help—to properly care for *both* my children.

With two teenagers and myself, we really needed a larger home than the small two-bedroom apartment Michaela and I had been living in, so Donna and I started praying for a home with enough space for all of us. We even made a list, which read something like this: Three bedrooms, two bathrooms, large kitchen, living room and finished basement area. I suggested we buy a townhouse, live in it for a few years until Elliot and Michaela finished school and then sell it and divide the profit. This all sounded great in theory, but when it came to providing the down payment, neither of us actually *had* any money! However, we did have a lot of faith in our new-found God (that He would supply all our needs). We also had ten dollars to put gas in my car to go house-hunting!

Within a few days we actually found a townhouse in Port Moody, which had every single item on our list. It also had a lower level which provided Donna with enough space for a bed-sitting room and storage. Donna and I managed to borrow the required amounts for our down payment, and with both our incomes we qualified for the mortgage. We became the proud owners of a three-bedroom townhouse. After that, we split every household expense one-third for Donna and two-thirds for me because I had the kids. It worked very well.

Following our move to Port Moody, I started attending the Port Moody Pentecostal Church. I had a strong desire to serve God in some way. When the pastor said he needed someone to type the weekly bulletin, I volunteered for the job. I was thrilled that once again, God had put me in the right place at the right time. Every Saturday morning for the next three years, I happily used my secretarial skills to type and photocopy the church bulletin.

There were quite a few single adults in the Port Moody congregation—more than enough to form our own Bible study group. Donna and I eagerly offered our home for the meeting place. One of the first to join the group was a woman named Gail. Being single mothers with teenagers, Gail and I had much in common and soon became close friends. Over the next few years, we supported each other through many trying times. A dedicated member of our group, Gail also generously opened up her home to many of our functions. She is now happily remarried and has three grandchildren.

It was at this Port Moody church that I sang my first solo. On the night I was to sing, Gail, Donna and Michaela gathered on the front row, to pray in earnest that all would go well. They had only heard me singing at home (I have always referred to myself as a *kitchen sink* singer). No one knew what would happen up at the pulpit with a microphone in my hand—myself included. All I knew for sure was that I loved to sing worship songs to my Saviour. My voice was a little shaky to start, but after the first few notes, it went quite well. Singing many more times after that did not lessen the stage fright. However, I did grow to enjoy *making a joyful noise unto the Lord* and no one seemed to notice my knocking knees.

During the years we lived in Port Moody, the townhouse was used for Bible studies, potluck suppers and many other events. Our home was a regular haven for visitors, especially Elliot and Michaela's friends. There was always room for one more at our table and we never went hungry.

Through many miraculous events, we obtained a washer and dryer, beds, drapes, and many other items to help us have a comfortable home and sense of security. God really did supply all our needs when we put our absolute trust in Him.

We lived out the message of Hebrews Chapter 13, without realizing it!

> *Keep on loving each other... Do not forget to entertain strangers, for by so doing some people have entertained angels without knowing it.*

Donna and I are two very different personalities. When we lived in Port Moody, she was into hiking, bike-riding and wool-weaving. I, on the other hand, was happy to stay at home, painting and decorating, learning worship songs, watching television or baking cookies. Numerous times, after hiking to the top of a local mountain, Donna would arrive home and be unable to resist joining me for tea and homemade cookies.

The school track beside our home provided a great place to exercise. Sometimes Donna would ride her bike around the track while I would walk. When she encouraged me to get more exercise, my cheeky answer was always, "Donna, you know whenever I feel like exercising, I just lie down until the feeling goes away!"

Donna, Michaela, Elliot and I lived together for almost four years. They were happy, productive years for all of us. Elliot and Michaela graduated from grade twelve and started working. Elliot took flying lessons and obtained his commercial pilot's licence for small planes. He also spent time in Ontario and Pakistan with Canada World Youth. Michaela successfully completed a hairdressing course and now owns and operates her own salon.

When the time was right, Donna and I sold the townhouse and divided our profit exactly as planned. Our home had been used for the Lord's work. We were satisfied and blessed.

~

As I grew in faith, my prayers often included the question, *"What is your plan for my life Lord?"* His answer to my prayers seemed to be *wait*—so I waited.

I became quite adept at juggling church, home and work. My job was demanding. However, despite an increasingly hectic lifestyle, the future looked rosy indeed.

I had a dream to build a cabin on my brother's acreage near Sorrento (in the picturesque Shuswap Lakes area of Central British Columbia) and started putting a little money aside to make the dream a reality.

It was during this time I experienced a slight loss of stamina and felt lightheaded when standing. At age fifty, I certainly didn't have the same physical abilities as Gail and Donna. The ritual of the Saturday afternoon nap came into being.

~

A Mosaic of Friends

Meeting Evelyn in August 1988 was quite by accident. I had decided, on my way home from work, to drop some boxes off at the apartment I had just rented in Coquitlam. It was a beautiful, sunny afternoon. Traffic, however, had backed up considerably in the five o'clock rush hour and by the time I turned onto the quiet street behind the apartment building, I was exhausted, and not in a very pleasant mood.

I was just about to get out of my car and tackle the boxes, when I saw an elderly woman on the sidewalk ahead of me struggling to carry groceries into the apartment building next door. For the next few minutes, I actually sat in my car arguing with God, telling Him in no uncertain terms just how hot, tired and miserable I felt. God wasn't giving me any sympathy, however, and I knew my conscience wouldn't rest until I offered some assistance. Wearily, and rather reluctantly, I got out of my car and walked over to where the woman was still struggling.

"Do you need some help?" I asked.

The relieved look on her face cheered me instantly. Together we carried about ten bags of groceries up the back steps of the building, opened the locked door, proceeded up more stairs and along a corridor to her front door.

Once inside, I was instantly impressed with the obvious cleanliness and order of the place. Beautiful china ornaments and birds were lined up along the top of the kitchen cupboards (how on earth did she get up there to clean them? I wondered). The furniture was immaculate French provincial and without a spec of dust. After placing all the grocery bags beside the dining table, I did something that would change both our lives forever. On the spur of the moment, I gave this stranger my phone number and offered to drive her to the grocery store whenever she needed to go again. As she looked up at me, her grey eyes twinkled, and straightening her shoulders somewhat, as if a huge load had just been removed from them—she accepted my offer.

Over the months and years that followed, our trips to the grocery store progressed into lunches out and wanderings around the mall, usually looking for new blouses. Evelyn loved to shop. She would go all day if I let her. It was always me who got tired first. She used to get mad because all I wanted to do was get home for a cup of tea. At the time, I was at a loss to figure out how an 85-year-old woman pushing a walker, had more energy than I did.

Evelyn had a special dream. She wanted to experience an Alaska Cruise. One day, we were browsing in the mall and she asked me to take her to the travel agent. A short while later, she had booked the trip and bought a new suitcase with wheels. I was concerned about her travelling alone. Much as I hate boats *and* water, I decided to accompany her. Our Alaska cruise became a very meaningful event for both of us. It gave Evelyn many fond memories to sustain her in the quiet years ahead. It helped me to put aside some of my fears.

That trip still provides us with plenty to talk and laugh about today. Evelyn still chuckles when she describes the look of horror on my face as the cruise ship left the dock in Vancouver.

In the winter months Evelyn didn't venture out too often, as she was afraid of slipping on icy streets and breaking something. I particularly remember one Christmas Evelyn and I were going to be alone on Christmas Day. We decided to have Christmas dinner together. I cooked a chicken and all the trimmings and carried the feast over to Evelyn's place in a laundry basket. As soon as she opened the door, I knew she had taken special care to dress up. Her silver hair was curled to perfection. She wore a beautiful mauve silk dress and dainty satin slippers. A picture of loveliness etched in my memory forever!

I am happy that our friendship is still going strong today. Evelyn is in a nursing home now. Since it's a fair distance to drive, I'm not able to visit her frequently. However, when we do get together, we are always able to take up right where we left off. I still enjoy hearing about her childhood, the depression years, and her life struggles. What a woman of courage she is!

I have learned so much from Evelyn over the years. She taught me to have compassion for the elderly. She knew all there was to know about being frugal (she had, after all survived the great depression) and encouraged me to save for the future. A woman of firm opinions, it was pointless arguing with her, so I eventually learned patience. It must be true what they say about age bringing wisdom, because Evelyn is one of the wisest people I know.

I'm glad I stopped to help her that day. I wouldn't have missed our time together for anything. One thing I can say for sure, our meeting was no accident!

Oh, and those beautiful china birds? It eventually became *my* chore to climb up on the step ladder to clean them!

~

I'd been living in the Coquitlam apartment for two years when Donna introduced me to her friend Cindy, who was interested in renting a house with someone. Cindy was studying at Simon Fraser University and hoping to become a teacher. I invited her over for coffee and we became instant friends. We decided to look for a house to rent in

Coquitlam, which would be close to my work and easy for Cindy to get to SFU. Noisy neighbours in my apartment building were driving me crazy. I longed for some peace and quiet.

We quickly found a main level, three bedroom suite in a house on Sprice Avenue in Coquitlam. We moved in a month later. A compassionate and dedicated Christian, Cindy had a desire to serve God and witness to others. Meeting her friends from university and getting to know her family was a great pleasure for me. The only unfortunate incident that occurred while we lived together was the fire!

We'd been living in the house about a year when I came home from work one afternoon to find the upstairs suite filled with thick grey smoke. Our neighbours had called the fire department and had smashed open the back door to let my cat out. When Cindy drove up the street a few minutes later, she was shocked to see our house surrounded by firemen, fire trucks and interested bystanders.

We were told the fire was caused by an electrical wiring problem in the basement suite. One of the firemen came up to me and said, "It's a miracle the windows didn't smash with the heat of the blaze."

Thankfully, we had insurance. Everything we owned was covered in a yellowish-grey film of greasy smoke-dust. The next day, all our furniture and possessions were packed up and taken away to be cleaned. Work began to rebuild the gutted basement suite and replace carpets, etc. upstairs.

Our landlord generously allowed us to live in the basement of his own home while the repairs were being completed. After a couple of months we moved back into the house but it no longer felt like home. A few months later we moved out. Cindy was able to share a house with some other students and I moved into the basement suite of a new house near the Coquitlam Centre.

Cindy and I kept in touch over the years. I attended her wedding. She and her husband Geoff recently moved to Pitt Meadows and we all attend Maple Ridge Alliance Church. We have a very special relationship. It's a great blessing for me to see them in church every Sunday with their beautiful daughter, Katherine.

One thing for sure, Cindy and I know what it's like to go through a *fire*!

~

I first met Janine when she came to one of the Bible study sessions at our townhouse in Port Moody. Janine has actually visited my hometown of Bournemouth and walked along the same beaches where I played as a child. This is just one of the special bonds between us.

Janine suffered much from a traumatic childhood in France. At sixteen she left her family home in Paris to work on a farm in England. She was only paid a minimum wage, but at least she had the opportunity to learn and practise the English language. She later returned to Paris to finish up her schooling. In 1949 she applied to several hospitals in southern England as she wanted to become a nurse. She was accepted at Basingstoke Mental Hospital. While in training, she met her future husband. They came to Canada in 1954 with their three-year-old son and settled in Northern Ontario.

Janine is no stranger to emotional or physical pain. Having endured three separate back injuries she has had a number of operations on her spine in an attempt to correct the problems. In almost constant pain, she uses a walker to navigate her apartment. However, with the use of a motorized scooter, she attends church and goes shopping.

Janine also holds Bible studies in her home. She never ceases to amaze me with her faith in God, courage and kindness of heart.

~

My friend Sandra loves gardening. Over the years we have spent many warm Sunday afternoons sitting in her beautiful back yard, sipping cool drinks and planning retirement strategies. Together with our friends Josie and Beryl, we make up our own version of *Steel Magnolias*. We have all experienced the pain of divorce, the struggle of raising children alone and the fight to keep our heads above water financially. We still get through the tough times by helping and supporting each other.

~

It was my friend Josie who encouraged me to keep up with my writing. She truly is a *woman of courage* who has experienced many trials in the past few years. When her daughter recently needed a bone marrow transplant to correct a serious blood disorder, Josie was there—cooking, cleaning, driving to the hospital and caring for her young grandson. No mother could have done more for their child. I was very proud of her.

Josie and I both emigrated to Canada from the U.K. in the sixties. We share many fond memories of the *old country*, have a grand sense of humour and are blessed with what we call *good old British spunk!*

~

Sharon and I first worked together in 1979. We were both single moms, working hard and trying to raise our children properly. Early in the friendship we made a pact. We promised each other we would never talk about mundane issues like the price of soap powder, etc. Today we are still the best of friends. Our topics of conversation range from politics, travel and world issues, to health, diet and exercise. I love Sharon's *no nonsense* approach to life and her rich, vibrant character.

~

Almut is also a longtime friend. She was my first supervisor at the bank in Maillardville. She taught me how to calculate *per diem* interest—something I have never forgotten. Now that we are both retired, we have fun going out together. A few months back, Almut took me to the Vancouver Art Gallery, which I enjoyed tremendously. Suppers together are great fun. We can talk for hours without stopping for breath. Almut's openness and honesty are the character traits I love most.

~

My friend Liz was a war bride. She first met her future husband John at The Greyhound pub in Croydon, Surrey, England. As a member of the Women's Royal Naval Service, she crossed the Atlantic by boat five times during the Second World War, taking care of other war brides and their babies who were destined for Halifax, Nova Scotia. After her sixth and final crossing in March 1945, accompanied by husband John, she stayed in Canada to start a new life in a new country. Liz and I both know what it's like to walk down the streets of a Canadian city and not know a single person. We are fiercely proud of both our English heritage and Canadian citizenship. We share many common bonds. Yes, we still love steak and kidney pie!

Friends Together

Olga and I have been friends for more than twenty-three years. She first took me under her wing when we worked together in 1978. She was the best bank teller I had ever known. Balancing to the penny was something she accomplished easily, year-in and year-out. When I had hardly any furniture, she helped me buy a new hide-a-bed for my living room. When it came to cooking, Olga introduced me to lasagna and pasta dishes and I introduced her to roast beef and Yorkshire pudding.

I visited with Olga just the other day. She insisted on being the first person to order and pay for a copy of this book. When I left, I gave her chapter one to read. Twenty minutes later I phoned to let her know I had arrived home safely.

I was shocked to hear her crying.

"What's wrong?" I asked. "Are you hurt?"

"I'm OK," she mumbled through her tears.

"What's wrong?" I asked again.

She managed to get a few words out. "Love chapter one... *sniff*... good story... *sniff*... made me cry."

I felt awful.

After much apologizing on my part and nose-blowing at her end of the phone, we started to laugh.

Dear, sweet, sensitive Olga. You may have bought the first book, but I think I'll have to read it to you in small doses—one page at a time!

Isn't that what friends are for?

CHAPTER SIX

The Sting Called Parkinson's

My whole body trembled as I pushed open the heavy glass doors of the medical building and forced myself to step outside into the afternoon sunshine. The neurologist's words echoed through my mind repeatedly; "Pauline, you have Parkinson's disease."

In a daze, I slowly walked back to the side street where I had parked my car just one hour earlier. People walked past me without noticing my inner turmoil. Mothers with children, elderly couples, professional people in a hurry—no one gave me a second glance. To them it was just another sunny afternoon in which to enjoy a stroll, buy flowers from the corner store, or visit someone in the hospital across the street. For me, however, nothing would ever be the same again. I remember thinking, "I'll never forget *this* day for the rest of my life."

The Invisible Thief

I have no recollection of *feeling* the original sting of Parkinson's disease. I'm unable to look at a calendar and tell you the day, month or year that dopamine-producing cells in the base of my brain started to die. I only know the disease began subtly and progressed gradually.

On looking back over the past few years, I realized there had been many physiotherapy treatments for muscle aches and pains that were very slow to heal. There were also numerous occasions I'd arrived home from work exhausted and fallen asleep watching the six o'clock news. Certainly, since my fiftieth birthday, I had noticed a definite drop in energy levels. I had never been that energetic (as any member of my family will tell you) but even *I* realized I had no pep. At the end of the day, all I longed for was that moment when my tired, aching muscles could be soothed in a warm bath.

After one particular physiotherapy session, I *did* notice it was much easier to swing my arms when walking the two blocks home, but didn't think this was important enough to make a big deal out of it. I still didn't think there was anything *seriously* wrong with me.

Everyone said, "It's just menopause." However, I wasn't totally convinced. Following numerous checkups and blood tests, my doctor was unable to find anything physically wrong, but I knew *something* had to be causing the fatigue. I was sick and tired of feeling sick and tired. Many times I told friends my body felt like it belonged to a ninety-year-old, but other than that, I thought perhaps I needed more rest (or hormones!) It almost seems as if the disease itself had tricked my brain into thinking *"it's just my age, or the stress I'm under at work, or if I get some more sleep this weekend, I'll feel better."*

~

The Reluctant Vacationer

As is often the case with diagnosis of Parkinson's disease, it was my family who sounded the alarm in August 1999.

In previous years I had spent many vacations with David and Margaret. When they retired to Sorrento, their country home provided the perfect place for relaxation. Every summer I gladly left the hectic city lifestyle behind for a couple of weeks, to recharge body and spirit. Some years, my vacations were carefully timed to coincide with goat birthing, so I could help with bottle feeding the baby goats. Everything about rural life intrigued me. I longed for the day when I could quit work and retire to the country. The office divider beside my desk was covered with scenic shots of Sorrento to remind me of my retirement dreams.

In recent years my niece Christine and nephew Stephen, together with their respective families, had also moved to Sorrento. Family suppers now involved cooking for anywhere between nine and sixteen people, depending on who was visiting at the time. Every year I looked forward to these family get-togethers with happy anticipation.

However the summer of 1999 was different somehow. I lacked my usual enthusiasm. The five-hour drive I used to enjoy now loomed ahead of me like an insurmountable barrier.

Not wanting me to miss out on a few days vacation, David traveled down to Vancouver on the bus, so that the next morning he could keep me company and share the driving on my planned trip to Sorrento.

David and I enjoyed the drive and Margaret was very happy to see us arrive safely. For the next few days I sat around reading, enjoying the fresh air, beautiful scenery and the company of my family.

I had no idea they were watching my every move.

Margaret had noticed my difficulty getting up from a chair and general lack of stamina. She mentioned to David that I appeared to be walking hesitantly—just like her friend Barb, who had been diagnosed with Parkinson's disease three years earlier. One evening, after watching me struggle to put some food on my fork and slowly bring it up to my mouth, they decided to take action on my behalf. Margaret began keeping a mental note of the symptoms she and David had observed.

By the end of the week I felt somewhat rested and assured everyone it would be perfectly safe to drive myself home.

Bad mistake!

By the time I reached Hope, I'd been driving for four hours and was totally exhausted. My arms and legs felt like unresponsive lumps of wood and I had absolutely no reserve of energy left. How I completed the last leg of the journey and reached home safely I will never know.

I felt lonely, scared and very tired. My physical weakness now forced me to acknowledge that something was very wrong.

That night Michaela phoned me and we had a long talk. She said, "Mom, if you *could know* what is wrong with you, would you *want* to know?"

"Yes, of course I would want to know." I replied.

"Well... Mom, I've been talking to Auntie Margaret and Uncle David and we think you may have something like Parkinson's disease."

I was very quiet after that. It's probably one of the few times in my life I've been speechless!

Michaela then filled me in on the telephone conversations she'd had with Margaret and David and how they had offered to drive down to talk to me in person because they didn't want me to be alone. When Michaela assured them she could handle the situation on her own, it was decided *she* would be the one to break the news to me.

After spending hours on the Internet retrieving all the information she could find on Parkinson's disease, my daughter took a deep breath and made the call.

Margaret called later that night and at her urging, I promised to go back to the doctor for more tests. Margaret told me she planned to fax a letter to my doctor first thing Monday morning, describing my symptoms. I begged her to wait until after my next appointment. Thank heavens she ignored me.

Bright and early Monday morning, David drove into Sorrento and faxed the letter. Within five minutes of receiving it, my doctor was on the phone (long distance) to Margaret and they had *'the talk'* that would ultimately bring the answer to all our questions.

I must admit, on previous visits to my doctor, all I ever told her was that I continually felt tired and my muscles ached. Since I was a relatively new patient, she hadn't had the opportunity to really be aware of any physical changes. However, being supplied with the additional information in Margaret's letter and having talked with her on the phone, my doctor was able to solve the puzzle quickly. She told Margaret she *had* noticed my lack of facial expression recently and promised she would make an appointment for me to see a neurologist. Two weeks later, he confirmed the diagnosis.

When my son Elliot heard the news, he asked if I felt afraid. In all honesty, I told him I was not afraid. On learning I had Parkinson's disease, I actually experienced a certain relief. Now, at last, I knew why I felt so tired! I could tell he had difficulty in fully realizing how I felt, but his hand on my shoulder and the concern in his eyes, spoke volumes.

Michaela still couldn't understand how she failed to notice the early symptoms. She comforted me by saying, "Don't worry Mom, I'll look after you." I was completely unprepared for this reversal in roles and tried to reject the idea. Thankfully, she's extremely patient where I'm concerned and allowed me some time to adjust. A few days later (for the first time in our adult lives) *she* accompanied *me* to the doctor's office.

Thus began stage one of my journey into the unknown realms of brain disease. Already I was hoping someone would discover a cure (next week would be nice!)

From the knowledge I have gained since my diagnosis by reading a myriad of books, magazines and articles on the subject, I'm certain I had Parkinson's disease for at least five years before I was diagnosed. The very early symptoms of muscular stiffness, slow movements and fatigue crept up on me slowly. By the time evidence of the disease became clearly visible, I had probably lost more than 70% of the dopamine-producing cells in a small but important part of my brain called the *substantia nigra*.

~

My neurologist started me on a gradually increasing dose of medication *(Sinemet CR)* which seems to have kept me fairly stable so far. Walking continues to be unsteady even with the medication and standing still for any length of time—such as in store lineups, causes me to feel lightheaded and extremely nervous. Even in my own home, I can only stand for short periods of time, so I take frequent rest breaks during the day and have learned to complete small tasks, such as peeling vegetables, sitting down.

At this time, the only side-effect I am experiencing from the drug is an increased frequency and intensity of dreams, which at the onset was extremely unnerving. Many nights I forced myself to stay awake until the early hours of the morning, hoping I wouldn't have another nightmare. I mentioned the dreams to my neurologist. He suggested I take half a pill in the evening, but this increased the early morning muscle stiffness. I finally settled on taking the last pill of the day half-an-hour earlier—at 8:30 p.m. instead of 9:00 p.m.—and put off going to sleep until after midnight.

I have also discovered reducing sugar intake in the evening (candies, chocolate, etc.) definitely gives me a more relaxed sleep. However, for an Englishwoman with a sweet tooth, this is the ultimate discipline!

Due to the complexities of the disease, I have learned from other Parkinsonians it can take quite a time to get properly diagnosed (anywhere from six months to two years). There are a number of other medical conditions which have similar symptoms to Parkinson's disease and these must first be ruled out.

The delay in recognizing *my* symptoms caused me to miss out on being able to apply for long-term disability benefits through my employer. In the Spring of '98, when I thought all I needed was a couple of months rest, I decided to accept *the offered* early retirement package, thinking I could easily get another job at some point in the future. Never in my wildest dreams did I envision a serious illness was about to raise its ugly head.

Right now, I'd like to offer a word of advice: If you know for sure you don't feel as well as you did last month or last year, please write down every one of your symptoms and show the list to your doctor. I am convinced it is of great benefit for the physician to see the whole picture and have more of a chance to put all the puzzle pieces together. It's great to have hindsight, but I sure wish I had known back in 1998 what I know today.

Some of the most common symptoms of Parkinson's disease are:

- **Bradykinesia** (slowness of movement).
- **Tremor**
- **Muscular rigidity**
- **Impaired balance**
- **Stooped posture**
- **Low blood pressure** (especially when standing)
- **Muscle cramps, soreness and fatigue**
- **Constipation**
- **Urinary frequency**
- **Bradyphrenia** (slowness of thinking)

Don't forget, if you feel unwell, there's always a reason! Also, ladies, when you reach your fifties, please don't glibly blame the menopause for every ill feeling—like I did.

~

I have recently discovered Parkinson's disease has some very strange aspects to it. For example, the skills I learned at a young age such as touch-typing, knitting, etc., I am still able to accomplish quite successfully (albeit slower than before). However, place a spatula in my hand and I no longer have the required dexterity to flip over a fried egg! It doesn't matter how long I stand in front of the stove willing my uncooperative hand to complete the action—I have to practically stand on my head to get an egg flipped around here! (I know, I probably shouldn't eat fried eggs, but I was raised to believe fried egg sandwiches are good for you.)

~

Being able to type is a real blessing. I never thought I would be thankful for my strict typing teacher who, back in 1960, used to rap the knuckles of any student caught glancing at the typewriter keys. She made us pound those keys without looking, 'till we could do it in our sleep!

I have also heard of Parkinsonians who can still play the piano beautifully, but have great difficulty doing up buttons, pulling on pants, etc. On one particularly shaky Sunday morning recently, I had to ask my friend Cindy to fix my blouse buttons in the Church parking lot.

Another recent challenge for me is to successfully place a sandwich into a zip-lock bag. In fact, any action that requires placing an item *inside* something else, is now difficult to master. PD has its mysteries. That's for sure.

I've experienced some emotional struggles since those early days, mainly with the frustration of not being able to do what I once did. Acceptance of the gradual progress of PD symptoms is no picnic either. However, even with the challenges of living with Parkinson's disease, my life is full and satisfying. Quite simply, I appreciate and value the people around me more than ever before. I have made some new friends and received much love and caring from the friends I've known for years. I regard every single moment of each day as a precious gift.

CHAPTER SEVEN

People and Pets

I've been a *pet person* for as long as I can remember. Family pets are a wonderful source of unconditional affection. I have always delighted in their company and laughed at their hilarious antics. The proven fact that they relieve stress and even lower blood pressure is a bonus.

In my family we were taught to be kind to animals at a very early age and to respect the fact they are totally dependent on us for their basic needs. Over the years we've had pets of all kinds; dogs, cats, birds, hamsters, mice, fish—even goats. The variety was endless and limited only by the amount of space we had at the time.

For the past eight years, I have shared my home with *Mitzi* a short-haired (somewhat aloof) tabby. I also recently adopted an outdoor stray I have named *Sterling.*

Mitzi has developed certain feline rituals over the years. She has this habit of sticking her head in the fridge every time I open the door. In the early morning when I'm stumbling around trying to get the cream for my coffee, she's got her head in the fridge looking for tuna. So I yell *"Back up cat"* and she nonchalantly turns around, stopping briefly to rub her cheek on the edge of the fridge door as she passes. When I put the tuna in her dish, she'll often turn her nose up at it and walk away. So then I yell, *"If you don't eat it, I'll give it to Sterling"* and immediately, she goes back to her dish and eats every last crumb!

Always curious, Mitzi used to be in the habit of sitting on the edge of the tub and watching me take a bath, until one day her paws slipped and she fell on top of me! We both yowled in terror, and I ended up with cat-claw puncture marks and bruises where she landed on my arm! Of course, it was short-sleeve weather at the time and for weeks afterwards, when people stared at my arm, I had to smile sweetly and say, "The cat fell in the tub!"

~

I call Sterling my *cat angel* because he showed up at just the right time to bring me out of the doldrums.

Shortly after my diagnosis I was sitting out on the patio (feeling a bit despondent) when I happened to notice clumps of silver-grey fur stuck to the vinyl padded cushion on one of the chairs. I figured a stray cat had been sleeping there at night, so I covered the seat of the chair with a blanket. I then put out a dish of fresh water and waited to see if the cat came back.

He returned every night, and I took pleasure in peaking through the blinds to see his silver-grey form curled up on the blanket. As time passed, however, I noticed he was getting thin and the fur on his tail had some bald patches. So I started leaving out a bowl of cat food every morning—to help improve his condition. He devoured that first bowl of food in seconds and every morning after that he sat on the chair, waiting patiently for his breakfast.

It took many months before Sterling would allow me to get close enough to pet him and I have yet to hear him purr, but if the food dish is empty, he'll sit outside my living room window and meow at me until I feed him.

One day, a couple of young racoons chased him away and ate his food. He came back about an hour later, meowing pathetically for a second helping, which of course I quickly provided.

Sterling still eats like there's no tomorrow, but he's filled out nicely and his fur is thick and glossy. In fact, he is so large now, even the racoons stay out of his way.

I have to confess—I wasn't much help with the wildlife situation recently. I forgot to put my glasses on one dark winter morning, and seeing a grey shape on the patio, I inadvertently gave Sterling's breakfast to a visiting racoon. It's a miracle I didn't try to pet it!

For me, looking after Sterling and gaining his trust has been a lesson in patience. Also, when I wake up in the morning and my muscles are stiff and sore, I now have the necessary motivation to get up, get moving and feed those darn cats!

By the way, if you want to know the *real* difference between a dog and a cat, the story goes something like this: When you go to bed at night a dog will sleep on your feet because it loves **you**! A cat will sleep on your feet at night because it loves your **bed**!

Now, I don't expect you to go rushing out and pay big money for a huge dog that's going to get under your feet and trip you up. Please use your common sense regarding size, breed, gender, etc. Don't forget all pets are a commitment and need to be cared for properly.

However, if your situation allows it, the joys of pet ownership can enrich your life tremendously.

CHAPTER EIGHT

Safety in Numbers

A few weeks after my diagnosis, I contacted the B.C. Parkinson's Disease Association for information about support groups. They put me in touch with the facilitator of the closest Parkinson's Support Group, which met in Maple Ridge—about a twenty minute drive from my home.

I attended my first support group meeting a short time later and must admit, I was terrified. Thankfully, a woman came and sat beside me and started talking to me, or I think I would have bolted out of the room! It was a very informative meeting. However, as a relative newcomer to the disease, a lot of the topics discussed were alien to me—not to mention *very disconcerting*.

I'm sorry to say, at that point in my life, my own fears made it very difficult for me to see beyond the disease!

Spring and summer passed quickly. I didn't attend any more meetings. The September meeting was fast approaching but I was still unsure about the whole thing. Was I ready or not? Almost a year had passed since my diagnosis and I was definitely feeling stronger emotionally. This time, when I got the phone call telling me the date and time of the next meeting, I was determined to go. I seem to remember hastily saying my shortest prayer—HELP!

'PD-Day' arrived and I was pleasantly surprised to see a familiar face at the entrance to the Activity Centre (the woman who sat beside me at the first meeting). We walked in together. It didn't take very long for me to feel at home with everyone present. From that point on, I am relieved and happy to report I was able to look around the room at this group of friendly, spontaneous people without seeing the disease at all. I believe God worked a miracle in my heart and mind that day.

I also began to realize it might be just as difficult for longtime PD sufferers to adjust to seeing newcomers in the group and be reminded of their own earlier, less troublesome stages.

I would like to encourage those of you who have never attended a support group meeting to please make the effort. The long-term benefits, I can guarantee, will far outweigh your initial nervousness.

I can honestly say with great affection, the members of the Maple Ridge Parkinson's Support Group are some of the kindest, most courageous people I have ever met. It would have been *my* loss if I had never got to know them. The truth is, we are all on this journey together. Regardless of what stage we are at, the quality of our journey can be greatly enhanced by helping each other along the way. There is much valuable information to be learned and shared. You *can* make a difference!

Getting Around Safely

When I'm out walking there are times when the sidewalk feels like the rolling deck of a ship beneath my feet. I worry about falling and hurting myself or the worse-case scenario of *freezing* when crossing the street. Recently I came up with the idea of printing some *Parkinson's Alert* cards containing a brief explanation of my condition with my son and daughter's names and phone numbers. I then placed a card in every jacket and coat pocket, just in case!

Parkinson's Alert!

My name is Pauline Neck.
I have a neurological disorder that may cause unsteady or hesitant walking.
In the event I should fall, or need assistance, please call:

____

It may seem insignificant, but having that small card in my pocket helps me to feel secure. If I *were* involved in an accident or mishap of some kind, someone would eventually find the card and call my son or daughter.

Most of these anxieties miraculously disappear when I have my eight-year-old granddaughter with me. Of course she doesn't know it yet, but when I hold her hand to cross the street, it's now more for *my* benefit than hers.

I recently learned a lesson in basic human kindness. Early one morning I decided the time had come to tell the cashier at my local grocery store the reason for my awkwardness in retrieving money from my purse. It was hard to swallow my pride. Thankfully, there were only a few people in the store. I assured her I was not hung over, or on drugs, but my hand-shaking was due to Parkinson's disease. To my surprise, she came around the counter and gave me a hug!

To make things easier for me, I usually go to the store early in the morning or late at night, when lineups are short. Last week I shared with the young woman in our local drug store postal outlet my reason for always coming in around eight o'clock at night. When I told her I had Parkinson's disease and experienced great difficulty standing in a line up, she was very understanding.

I have found, once people know about your health challenges, they show a kindness and caring that otherwise might not have occurred. Parkinson's disease certainly brings out the best in people.

If you happen to be newly diagnosed and nervous about sharing your condition, I would recommend telling someone you are comfortable with (perhaps your hairdresser or barber). The first time is the hardest, but if you persevere it gets easier every time. Most of the people I regularly see around town know I have Parkinson's disease. It brings me much comfort to know that when I'm out and about, there are people who know my condition and if I needed assistance, they would help me.

I'm sure the days ahead will hold many more small victories and moments of pure joy. Like the other day when Hayley came bounding into the kitchen to tell me, "Grandma, it's five o'clock—time to take your pill!"

CHAPTER NINE

Women and Words

When I retired from my secretarial job, I acquired a computer, printer, desk and other accessories. At the time, I had no thoughts of writing a book. I was all set to join the ranks of other home-based businesses by providing word processing services. However, that particular dream (like the cabin in Sorrento) was not meant to be.

I joined the Port Coquitlam (British Columbia) Women and Words support group for writers in the Fall of 1998. At first, I felt awkward and out of place among such talented women. Gradually, however, their friendship and total acceptance helped me to relax. As I watched, listened and learned, I dared to believe someday I too would become a writer. For the longest time I was too nervous to share my efforts with the group, but once I started, there was no looking back! Somewhere along the way, shyness was replaced with a confidence I never knew I possessed.

My interest in writing began in the mid-seventies when I had the opportunity to set the type for a local history book and an autobiography. However, it wasn't until 1984 that I began to write poetry. In the Spring of 2000, writing became a daily occurrence and I slowly came to the realization I had an important message to share.

Today the members of *Women and Words* are very enthusiastic in their support of one another and daring to push ahead with their own writing goals. I think we all agree the group provides a safe haven for our work to be confidently shared, gently critiqued, and carefully edited. It is also a place where we learn from each other and encourage each other's talent and potential.

Of course, the ladies have all heard me moan in anguish when my writing instructor Norm advises me yet again, I'm writing *"too polite."* I must admit, I sometimes feel like a struggling fish at the end of his fishing line. I'm hooked on writing. From time-to-time I even delude myself into thinking I can swim away on my own, only to be pulled back to reality with his admonitions of *"tight, tight, tight. Cut, cut, cut."*

On a recent Saturday morning, however, I was the recipient of a genuine miracle in the form of the brilliant and delightful Carmen. As most of the ladies were attending a seminar, she was the only person to show up at my apartment. Carmen kindly offered to help me by editing the introduction to this book. Holding a bright yellow marker like an artist's brush, she creatively highlighted, deftly moved text, carefully deleted and transformed my somewhat mundane jumble of words into beautiful flowing, coherent sentences. "Did you hear that Norm—*flowing sentences?"*

I have to say this once and for all; I can't help writing like a polite, friendly Englishwoman. I *am* a polite, friendly Englishwoman. *(Proud Canadian citizen for more than thirty years—and still have the English accent.)*

Norm's latest request for more dramatics goaded me into

writing this poem. (Sincere apologies to any English women reading this.)

An Englishwoman's Lament

British reserve is a terrible thing,
"Stiff upper lip and all that."
Writing this book is really a stretch;
I'd much rather talk to the cat!

"Onward and upward," you say with aplomb!
My goodness, you are so brave.
I'd much rather ride in a black limousine,
And once in a while give a wave.

If it wasn't for people urging me on,
I'm sure I'd have long ago quit!
But there must be a bit of old Churchill in me,
So I'll not stop 'till the book's a big hit!

Individual talent in our *Women and Words* group is flourishing. Jackie has appeared in two local plays. Tara is teaching *The Virtues Project* (an innovative program created to build integrity and confidence in children and parents). Among her many creative talents, Lyn has self-published a number of books. She's also started *her* autobiography and has helped me with ideas for a book cover design. Ann writes beautiful poetry and is a great motivator. Lillian, our honourary member, thrills us with her action-packed short stories. Carmen recently attended a three-day publishing/editing seminar. Her science fiction writing keeps us all on the edge of our seats. Halia has just finished a story for children, and is also taking drama classes. Creatively, we are all very different, but that's what makes things interesting. We are unique, yet we all have the same drive.

After all, we could be doing other mundane things, like laundry, shopping or housework. Who in their right mind would want to, though, when all these ideas are flooding the brain? As it is, most of us have to plan our lives very creatively just to get computer time.

A Writer's Heart

Ah, the writer of words.
A gentle, tenderhearted soul
with a gift that cannot remain hidden
but must be shared.
Magical words to inspire, encourage,
excite and entertain.

No lid can snuff out the light of this candle,
even though it may flicker and dim;
when least expected, it bursts to life again.
A thought, when written down,
becomes a sentence, then a paragraph
and finally a chapter.

Even though many times we are rejected,
or just plain ignored;
that creative flame lights itself again,
with renewed hope and vigor.
This time, someone, somewhere, will enjoy
what we have written.

Removing the Sting

With toughened skins and spirits raised,
once more we venture forth into the unknown.
Fingers flying over computer keys,
ideas flooding the brain faster than
we can type them.

We are writers, and we are just beginning...

~

The reason we spend hours sitting staring at a computer screen is simple—we love to write. We're all hooked on the joy, the magnificent feeling that comes when we read back a sentence that is so perfectly, amazingly right. Apart from the discomfort of stiff shoulders and sore wrists when I happen to sit too long at this desk, writing has certainly given me great joy. The first time a Parkinson's magazine printed one of my poems, I was ecstatic! For days I had this silly grin on my face that nothing could erase.

~

As family and friends comforted me with their love and support, I again asked God for direction—gently reminding Him that I could no longer afford the luxury of waiting. His answer came loud and clear... *WRITE!*

In the months following my diagnosis, I jotted down ideas for keeping a positive attitude. I listed coping strategies and enjoyable activities. I wrote about the benefits of support groups, pet ownership, gardening, cooking, writing, singing—everything I could possibly think of to encourage myself to live life to the fullest, regardless of the difficulties I was experiencing. This therapeutic exercise was done not just for myself, but with the idea in mind that somehow I may be able to help other people facing similar situations.

I discovered there were many actual *blessings* from having Parkinson's disease, and wrote about them. I developed a deeper relationship with God and began trusting Him and thanking Him for every precious day.

Renewed in spirit and blessed with a strong faith, I began reaching out to others with words of inspiration and encouragement. When my Bible study leader asked me to share a poem with the group, I went home and wrote a new one. That's how this whole thing started—with one poem.

A Parkinsonian's Prayer

I wrote *All Our Days Belong to the Lord* in March 2000. The poem was originally written to encourage some of the members of my Bible study group who were also going through a particularly difficult time. On a personal level, the words of the poem became my own *Parkinsonian's prayer*.

ALL OUR DAYS BELONG TO THE LORD

Please give to me good length of days
in which to do your will.
Some days for singing songs of praise,
some days to just be still.

Lord, grant me courage to go on
and willing hands to serve.
Be patient with my anxious thoughts
and fill my heart with love.

When trouble comes upon me
and life's an uphill climb;
Help me surrender to your love
and feel your hand in mine.

For there's no doubt I need you,
without you I am lost.
Help me to lay my burdens
upon your rugged cross.

And when at last I see you,
and look into your face,
I'll lift my hands up to the one
who saved me by His grace.

In the months that followed, *All Our Days Belong to the Lord* appeared in both the S.W. Ontario and Quebec Parkinson's magazines and was also accepted for publication by the International Library of Poetry in their book *As Minutes Turn to Hours.*

The poem has been shared in churches, Bible studies and various support groups in B.C. with copies also being sent to people living in England, USA, Australia, New Zealand, Russia and Mexico. The response to the poem has been extraordinary, with many people saying the words were *just for them.*

My nephew's wife Robin recently created a lovely melody for these words and hopes to put it on a CD one day.

CHAPTER TEN

The Second Sting

And when you stand praying, if you hold anything against anyone, forgive him, so that your Father in heaven may forgive you your sins. *~Mark 11:25*

On a recent Sunday afternoon, some of the family came to my place for a visit. David and Margaret had driven down from Sorrento, to spend a few days with me. They had brought with them an old suitcase full of family photographs so I could pick out the ones I needed for this book.

It was a wonderful get-together. Elliot, Gosia and my grandson Maxwell had arrived. Michaela and Hayley also stopped in for a visit. My small living room was packed.

Michaela and Hayley were having fun going through the photographs and the rest of us were talking. I was in the kitchen, making tea. Michaela picked up a piece of paper from out of the suitcase and started reading. All of a sudden, she called out to me, "Mom, I didn't know your dad had Parkinson's disease."

The room was totally quiet as every eye turned toward me.

I stood there dumfounded and in shock. My dad had

Parkinson's disease? Why hadn't anyone told me?

A million thoughts ran through my mind. My emotions ran wild, giving me that queezy feeling like when a vehicle you're travelling in is going too fast, but there's nothing you can do about it. Someone brought me into the living room. I sat down and tried to compose myself.

Unfortunately, Michaela hadn't realized she had picked up a copy of an old letter from my sister, written to our half-brother Michael. In the letter she had conveyed the news of Dad's death. It turned out Dad hadn't contacted his second family for a number of years and Michael had written to my sister asking if she knew the whereabouts of his father. When Pat wrote to Michael, she had also sent a copy of the letter to David and Margaret and it was this copy that ended up in the suitcase of old photographs.

Pat was the only one who had visited Dad on a regular basis and had even brought him to Canada for a vacation in 1980. In his later years, she visited him in various nursing homes on the Isle of Wight and kept us informed of his situation. When Dad was dying, David flew to England to see him one last time and stayed with Pat to help her with the funeral arrangements.

Dad died in a nursing home on the Isle of Wight in 1988. He was seventy-seven years old. Looking back, I must have known about his various illnesses but in all honesty probably didn't care enough at the time to think twice about it. David and Pat hadn't remembered about Dad's Parkinson's disease either—until I was diagnosed, and then, out of concern for my feelings, had tried to shield me from finding out. However, had I been cognizant of the facts, I would certainly have talked to my doctors about Parkinson's disease years ago.

Filled with indignation, I ranted and raved for quite a

while. How could this man I had spent most of my life despising, still be able to hurt me when he'd been dead for years? This person, who had never (in my eyes) had the guts to be a real father, had been successfully blamed for just about everything that had ever gone wrong in my life. Now I had to deal with the knowledge that I had possibly inherited Parkinson's disease from *him*!

When I had calmed down a little, I realized, once again, God had been preparing me to receive this shocking news. Just three weeks earlier, the topic for the Sunday sermon at my church had been *forgiveness* and I had gone forward for prayer at the end of the service because I felt I was still holding onto some deep-rooted hostility toward my dad. One of the young women in the worship team prayed with me and I felt a definite release afterwards.

Now it felt as if the old wound had been viciously opened up again and the pain of the situation overwhelmed me. How on earth was I going to deal with this?

After everyone had gone home and I was alone with my thoughts, I phoned my friend Sandra to talk it all out. The next night I phoned Almut and talked it all out again—thank heavens they're good listeners! At Wednesday evening Bible study I shared the story yet again and asked for prayer. Then on the Friday morning, I turned on my radio, as usual, to listen to Charles Stanley and the miracle happened! Not only was he talking about forgiveness, but gave simple, explicit instructions on what to do if the person you needed to forgive was no longer living. *I took notes*!

At the end of the program, I sat on my couch and placed a photo of my dad on the loveseat across from me. With tears pouring down my face, I proceeded to berate him with every incident that had caused me to suffer hurt, pain and rejection (this went on for quite a while). Finally, the tears subsided and I told my dad that because Jesus had forgiven me of *my* sins, I, in turn, must now willingly forgive him of all the hurts he had caused, including this last, most vicious *sting*. Once again, I had to say the words out loud. *"Dad, I forgive you for everything. I believe you loved me and did what you thought was best for me at the time. I'm sorry you got Parkinson's disease."* I then got up from the couch and gently placed my dad's photograph back in its envelope.

Thank you, Charles Stanley. Your lesson on forgiveness helped me to move forward in freedom and have the ability to write this chapter without shedding one tear.

By a miracle of God's power, I am now able to think of my dad with love and compassion.

CHAPTER ELEVEN

Content to be Blessed

Keep your lives free from the love of money and be content with what you have, because God has said,

"Never will I leave you;
Never will I forsake you."

~Hebrews 13:5

When days are difficult and my brain isn't kicking in until at least five minutes *after* I've said something really stupid (happens to me *all* the time!) it helps to consider those things that really bring me contentment. I'm not talking about material gain such as cars, houses or expensive toys—which, by-the-way, can never bring you lasting happiness. I'm referring to those occasions when you wish time could stand still just for a few seconds longer, so the moment can be truly enjoyed to the fullest.

Thinking about these treasured moments, special events and things I'm thankful for, I came up with the following list—in random order, as the thought entered my mind. Your list may be quite different to mine, but I think you will be able to relate to most of the following:

- Hearing the words "I love you Mom."
- Reading stories to my grandchildren.
- Sipping coffee early in the morning and watching the sunrise.
- Saturday morning telephone chats with my sister.
- Evening telephone chats with my brother and sister-in-law.
- Special suppers with my family in Sorrento.
- Seeing snowdrops for the first time after a long winter.
- Receiving a surprise gift from my son-in-law.
- Photo's that catch my best side and don't show too many wrinkles.
- Listening to my cat purr as she sits beside me.
- Enjoying other people's cooking.
- Quality time spent with family and friends.
- Watching my children grow up into beautiful, caring adults.
- Answered prayers.

When I wake up each morning and I'm still breathing, I give thanks. When I can get out of bed, and shuffle to the bathroom without hitting my arm on the door, I know its going to be a good day!

~

My latest positive discovery involves swimming. My daughter and son-in-law recently moved to a house with a backyard pool and I was waiting for a warm day to try it out.

On a beautiful day in early July, I carefully stepped down into the water, and was pleasantly surprised by the immediate freedom of movement. No longer bothered with the balance problems of PD, I tried swimming a few strokes.

My muscles were definitely weak, so I just relaxed, gently moving my hands and arms to stay afloat.

In the water, I felt normal—free from the pull of gravity and the slow, hesitant walk I had come to accept as my lot in life. The swimming pool—a place of terrifying fear in childhood, now offered me the luxury of instantly feeling ten years younger!

What joy, to be free from all the weight of the world around me. I stayed in the water as long as possible, floating, paddling, stretching my muscles, totally enjoying myself and never wanting to return to land again. Of course, eventually my hands turned white and I had to get out (those first few steps on land felt like I had lead boots on).

I'm very careful to stay in the shallow end with my granddaughter, but one day soon, I'm going to ask my daughter to teach me to swim properly again.

Auntie Bee, I hope you're looking down on us and smiling.

~

The Blessings of Parkinson's

Toward the end of my working career, time management was a definite inconsistency with me and a constant challenge. My energy levels seemed to fluctuate from *medium* to *nil* and I had no idea why.

Now that I know I have Parkinson's disease, I am learning to think ahead and plan my days more efficiently. I find I must allow myself about double the length of time previously required for such necessities as bathing, hair washing, dressing and makeup. Since *rushing* and Parkinson's don't mix, I've discovered the extra time allowances have resulted in *eventual punctuality!*

I'm getting much better at judging just how much I can accomplish in one day energy-wise (except for the bread dough adventure). My friends now accept the fact I can only handle one major activity per day. Also, because I don't have the stamina to keep returning to the grocery store for *things forgotten,* I now make shopping lists. My sister-in-law has been trying to get me to do this for years.

Parkinson's also seems to have produced a bravery and a confidence that I've never experienced before. Following my diagnosis, I was consumed with the desire to make every moment of the rest of my life totally meaningful!

Late one night, I was reading a back issue of Reader's Digest, when a line written by William Shakespeare, ***Sweet are the uses of adversity***, leapt off the page and hit me right between the eyes! Instantly, I knew I'd found one of the solutions to *removing the sting* of Parkinson's disease. All I had to do was discover a way to *use* my adversity to help others.

The poem *All Our Days Belong to the Lord* was one of my first attempts to bring comfort and inspiration through the written word. The positive response to this poem has been a great encouragement to me personally.

Of course, I still experience moments when doubts wash over me like a flood. At these times the oddest thoughts pop into my mind, such as, "*suppose all I'm fondly remembered for is my Christmas candied nut recipe?*" At times like these, I wonder why on earth I am trying to write this book. Then out of the blue, someone will be encouraged or helped by something I have written and convince me I must keep going. When these positive experiences occur, I am renewed, strengthened and determined to carry on. Sometimes, when the topic is painful, I can only write a few lines a day. At other times, I can write for hours. Through it all, the desire to use my own particular adversity to help others is incredibly strong.

Once again, words written many years previously, when I was a new Christian, confirmed that God indeed has a special plan for my life, and will instruct and guide me along the way:

Quietly, so quietly,
the Spirit of God will come,
to prompt you into doing things
that otherwise would remain undone.
The gentle words to help a friend,
the kindness that abounds;
the love we show to others,
helps them to turn around—and find peace.

The ultimate blessing of Parkinson's continues to be a closer walk with God and a greater desire to serve Him. The realization that He continues to pour creative thoughts and ideas into this *slightly damaged* brain of mine, is a constant source of delight.

CHAPTER TWELVE

Living Today with Hope for Tomorrow

Therefore do not worry about tomorrow,
for tomorrow will worry about itself.
Each day has enough trouble of its own.
~Matthew 6:34

When I look toward the future, I think about all the research scientists and medical personnel who are on the front lines of the battle against Parkinson's disease. Their dedication and hard work will, I'm sure, result in many breakthroughs, new drugs, and ultimately a long-awaited cure.

With public consciousness and financial support on the increase, I'm confident the war against Parkinson's disease will be won. Of course, those of us who are struggling with the disease today, are hopeful a cure will be found very soon.

So what shall we do while we're waiting?

At this point in time, I can only share with you what works for me at my own particular stage of this life journey.

I pray, sing, read, laugh, joke and spoil myself as much as possible. When I'm feeling despondent, I try very hard to remember my own recipe for getting out of the doldrums:

Phone a friend,
pet a dog,
make a person smile.
Do something for others,
you'll feel better in a while.

If you are physically able, some of the suggestions listed below may also be of help to you:

- Go for a walk in a park or by the ocean—take a neighbor or friend with you.
- Continue with or take up an activity you enjoy: painting, writing, gardening, etc.
- Join an Activity Centre. There's always lots of fun things going on.
- Spend quality time with children and grandchildren.
- Buy flowers for yourself at least once a month.
- Join your local library.
- Rent movies.
- Attend Church. It's a comforting place to be on a Sunday morning.

More Suggestions:

When you don't feel like cooking supper, invite a friend over and order in. Those of your friends who are still working will also enjoy not having to cook. Some of my friends are employed in high stress jobs and enjoy winding down and having someone to laugh, joke and share the events of their day with.

Removing the Sting

When I'm having a good (sufficient energy) day I have discovered preparing a simple meal and sharing it with a friend brings me a lot of happiness. It's a pleasurable, relatively inexpensive way for me to show my appreciation.

I'm very fortunate that my daughter Michaela is a hairdresser, so whenever I need a little pick-me-up, she is always willing to shampoo, cut or perm my hair for me. Being around her is a delight and I love having beautiful hair.

I visit a chiropractor once a month. He works on my joints to keep them as supple as possible. He also massages my stiff muscles. As well as being a really caring person, he has the gift of making his patients feel better just by chatting with them. In addition, he's a wealth of information on alternate therapies and exercises.

Keeping flexible is a continuous battle nowadays, so I try to do as much gentle stretching exercise as I can. I prefer to exercise to praise music, that way I'm uplifting my spirit as well as exercising my body.

~

At this point in time, it helps me keep a positive outlook if I try to focus on the things I *can* do, rather than the things I can no longer do. This is where the tulips come in.

In August 2000, my friend Sandra gave me some tulip bulbs to plant in the pots on my patio. In true PD style, I put off doing anything with them until late January. Then, on a cold, rainy day, just for something to do, I grabbed a tablespoon from the kitchen drawer, went out to the patio, dug a few holes in the soil-filled pots, placed the tulip bulbs in the cold, wet earth, covered them over and went back indoors.

Over the next few weeks I forgot about the bulbs. Then

as the days started getting warmer, I noticed some green shoots poking up out of the soil. Every week the shoots grew a little bigger. Finally, the tulip buds appeared and blossomed into the most beautiful, delicate shade of pink tulips I have ever seen.

The tulips have been replaced with other plants now, but I keep a photograph of them on my kitchen shelf as a constant reminder that, *"As long as the earth endures, seedtime and harvest, cold and heat, summer and winter, day and night will never cease."* (Genesis 8:22).

~

Finally, please try to keep your sense of humour (if you can't find anything to laugh at, there's always yourself). For an example, I'll tell you all about my bread dough adventure, which took place on a sunny afternoon last summer. My Wednesday morning Bible study was just about over when we were notified that a number of surplus boxes of bread dough had been donated to the Church. When asked for a show of hands as to who would like to take a box, I put my hand up! One of the ladies kindly carried the box of dough and placed it on the front seat of my car.

When I arrived home, I realized the box was too heavy to lift out of the car all at once. I would have to divide the dough in half. I went up to my apartment and got a large bowl and a knife. So there I was, leaning over the front seat, cutting up clumps of dough and dropping them into a bowl to carry upstairs. Thankfully, I made the two trips back to the apartment without anyone seeing me.

As it was a warm, sunny day, I decided my south-facing picture-window sill would be the perfect place to let the dough rise. There was an awful lot of dough, but I carefully cut it into pieces and formed rolls and small loaves. I put them in greased pans on the window sill and went out for coffee. When I got back to my apartment a couple of hours later, there was raised dough all over the place, and I spent the next five hours (with many rest breaks in between) baking bread!

~

I try to look on the bright side. My King James Bible teaches, "A merry heart doeth good like a medicine." (Proverbs 17:22)

Of course, having a grand sense of humour can be both a blessing or a curse. Now that I have Parkinson's disease, I have a tendency to speak first and think later. Most of the time people know I'm joking and take my comments lightly, but often there's a very fine line between humour and sarcasm, so I must be careful.

My friend Susan and I now have an agreement to forgive each other in advance for anything we might say that could cause offense. I am very thankful for Susan. She is the woman who sat beside me at my very first Parkinson's support group meeting.

Susan and I share our love for God and concern for family. When I'm having a difficult day, or trying to write about a particularly painful incident, I know I can phone her and she will help me through it. We recently discovered both of us have fax machines, so now whenever I write a new poem, I fax it over to her. Susan is another kindred spirit who understands adversity all too well.

~

When I look back and see all the special people God has placed in my life to help me, I am humbled by His loving protection. I think of my sister, who at twelve years old, hid from the school inspector, so she could stay home and look after me. She has continued to show her love and caring in so many ways over the years.

Auntie Bee took a frail, angry, seven-year-old into her heart and home.

My brother David, also generously provided a secure, loving home and family for me, without ever counting the cost. He has watched out for me my whole life.

Margaret, my dear sister-in-law, whose strength, wisdom and love have been a blessing to me for as long as I can remember.

My amazingly talented and caring children and grandchildren, whose unconditional love sustains me—even in the darkest hours.

Evelyn, my friend for over thirteen years now, has shared her vast knowledge and life experiences with me and taught me all about compassion.

Donna, my dear friend and kindred spirit, whose words of comfort always strengthen and uplift me.

My many kind and supportive friends—especially Sandra, Josie, Olga, Almut, Sharon, Liz, Lynn, Janine, Maureen, Gail, Berna and Faye.

The wonderful group of people who make up my church family and Bible study partners—who have been so faithful in their loving prayer support over the years.

The members of the Maple Ridge Parkinson's Support Group and Sandy & friends at PLWP. Their friendship and encouragement has been a great blessing to me.

And the idea for this book would never have blossomed without the inspiration and encouragement from the lovely ladies at *Women and Words*.

Then there are the friends I manage to see or talk to just

a few times a year, and the talented group of people I worked with for more than twenty years.

Like precious gems in a jeweled crown, each one of my friends enhances and beautifies the other. Whether it's Sandra's quiet strength and integrity, Josie's humour and compassion, Almut's kindness and generosity or Sharon's thoughtfulness and honesty, each one of them is a true blessing. We laugh together, cry together, encourage and help each other along the way. I am very thankful for each one of them.

~

No one really knows for sure what tomorrow will bring. All we can do is live today to the best of our ability with God's help and guidance. As we place our trust in Him, we receive an abundance of *"peace that passes all understanding."*

I believe God's promise that He will never leave me nor forsake me. I was definitely a lost sheep and my Lord, in His infinite grace and mercy welcomed me back to the fold.

It is God who fills me with hope for the future. I know He will look after me until that day when I can look into my Saviour's face ... *and lift my hands up to the One who saved me by His grace.*

For however many days are ordained for me (only God knows), I plan on continuing to embrace my faith, love my family and enjoy the company of good friends.

~

A Prayer from the Heart

Help me give thanks to you Lord,
even when I don't feel like it.
Let me sing praises to you, all the day long.
Make my sleep sweet and may I dream
only of your loving kindness.
Grant that I may bring glory to your name,
for you truly are good
and your love endures forever and ever. Amen

Appendix

Sources of Public Information

Parkinson Society Canada
Société Parkinson Canada

Mission Statement:
Parkinson Society Canada/Société Parkinson Canada is the national voice of Canadians living with Parkinson's. Our purpose is to ease the burden and find a cure through advocacy, education, research and support services.

National Office and Regional Partners

PSC National Office
4211 Yonge Street, Suite 316
Toronto, Ontario. M2P 2A9
Phone: (416) 227-9700
Toll Free: (800) 565-3000
Fax: (416) 227-9600
www.parkinson.ca

The Parkinson's Society of Alberta
Edmonton General, Room 3Y18
11111 Jasper Avenue
Edmonton, Alberta. T5K 0L4
Phone: (780) 482-8993
Toll Free: (888) 873-9801
Fax: (780) 482-8969

www.parkinsonalberta.ca
The Parkinson's Society of Southern Alberta
480D - 36th Avenue S.E.
Calgary, Alberta. T2G 1W4
Phone: (403) 243-9901
Toll Free (Alberta): (800) 561-1911
Fax: (403) 243-8283
www.parkinsons-society.org

Saskatchewan Parkinson's Disease Foundation
Box 102, 103 Hospital Drive
Saskatoon, Saskatchewan. S7N 0W8
Phone: (306) 966-8160
Fax: (306) 966-8030

PSC Manitoba Region
825 Sherbrook Street, Suite 204
Winnipeg, Manitoba. R3A 1M5
Phone: (204) 786-2637
Fax: (204) 975-3027

Ontario Division:
PSC Central & Northern Ontario Region
4211 Yonge Street, Suite 316
Toronto, Ontario. M2P 2A9
Phone: (416) 227-9700
Toll Free National: (800) 565-3000
Fax: (416) 227-9600

PSC Southwestern Ontario Region
4500 Blakie Road, Unit #117
London, Ontario. N6L 1G5
Phone: (519) 652-9437
Toll Free Ontario: (888) 851-7376
Fax: (519) 652-9267

Parkinson's Society of Ottawa-Carleton
1053 Carling Avenue
Ottawa, Ontario. K1Y 4E9
Phone: (613) 722-9238
Fax: (613) 722-3241
www.parkinsons.ca

La Société Parkinson du Québec
1253 McGill College, Suite 402
Montreal, Quebec. H3B 2Y5
Phone: (514) 861-4422
Toll Free: (800) 720-1307 - National Francophone line
Fax: (514) 861-4510
www.infoparkinson.org

PSC Maritime Region
5475 Spring Garden Road, Suite 407
Halifax, Nova Scotia. B3J 3T2
Phone: (902) 422-3656
Toll Free (NS, NB & PEI): (800) 663-2468
Fax: (902) 422-3797

PSC Newfoundland / Labrador Region
P.O. Box 2568, Stn. C
St. John's NF A1C 6K1
Phone: (709) 754-4428
Toll Free (NFLD / Labrador): (800) 567-7020
Fax: (709) 754-5868

B.C. Parkinson's Disease Association

Mission Statement:
The B.C. Parkinson's Disease Association exists to address the personal and social consequences of Parkinson's disease through education, outreach, scientific research and public awareness.

B.C. Parkinson's Disease Association
890 West Pender Street, Suite 600
Vancouver, B.C. V6C 1K4
Phone: 604-662-3240
Toll Free: (BC only): 1-800-668-3330
Fax: 604-687-1327
E-mail: info@parkinson'sbc.com
www.parkinson'sbc.com

Victoria Epilepsy and Parkinson's Centre Society
813 Darwin Avenue
Victoria, B.C. V8X 2X7
Phone: (250) 475-6677
Fax: (250) 475-6619
www.vepc.bc.ca

American Parkinson Disease Association

Mission Statement:
The American Parkinson Disease Association, Inc. (APDA) provides educational, referral and support programs to medical professionals, patients, their families and the public at large through regional symposia, educational literature and video tapes. APDA has 64 Chapters and more than 800 support groups; funds 58 Information & Referral Centers and sponsors research on Parkinson's disease by funding Advanced Centers for Parkinson Research, Fellowships and Research grants.

American Parkinson Disease Association
1250 Hylan Boulevard
Suite 4B
Staten Island
New York 10305-1946
Phone: 1-800-223-2732
Fax: 718-981-4399
E-mail: info@apdaparkinson.org
www.apdaparkinson.org

Parkinson's Disease Society of the United Kingdom

The Society's Mission Statement:
The Parkinson's Disease Society of the United Kingdom (PDS) works with people who have Parkinson's, their families and carers, and health and social care professionals. The mission of the PDS is the conquest of Parkinson's and the alleviation of the suffering and distress it causes through research, education, welfare and communication.

Parkinson's Disease Society of the United Kingdom
(Registered Charity Number 258197)
215 Vauxhall Bridge Road, London SW1V 1EJ
Tel: 020-7931-8080 Fax: 020-7233-9908
E-mail: enquiries@parkinsons.org.uk
www.parkinsons.org.uk
Helpline (freephone): 0808-800-0303 [Available Monday-Friday (except Bank Holidays), 9:30 am-5:30pm]

Some Very Special Books

These are just a few of the books that have profoundly influenced my thinking *and writing* over the years:

- The King James and NIV Bibles.
- Love is Letting Go of Fear *by Gerald G. Jampolsky, M.D.*
- Tough Minded Faith for Tender Hearted People *by Robert H. Schuller*
- How to Live Like a King's Kid *by Harold Hill with Irene Harrell.*
- I Work With Angels *by Rev. Edward W. Oldring.*
- Today and For Life *by Bernice Gerard.*
- All I Really Need to Know I learned in Kindergarten *by Robert Fulghum.*
- The Happiest People on Earth
  The personal story of Demos Shakarian, founder of The Full Gospel Business Men's Fellowship International. As told to John and Elizabeth Sherrill.
- Too Tough to Cry, A True Story of Suffering and Redemption *by Paul Powers.*

To learn more about Parkinson's disease, I would recommend reading The Parkinson's Handbook *by Dwight C. McGoon, M.D.*

Author's Note

Now that the book is finished, and I can relax, I thought I would have a little fun and share some humorous banter (just like they do at the end of some television shows). So, why don't you put the kettle on, make a pot of tea, grab a couple of cookies and prepare to spend a few lighthearted moments with me.

First of all, there are some awards to present: *Good listener* awards go to all my friends and relatives, but especially Michaela and Frank, Elliot and Gosia, my sister Pat, brother David, sister-in-law Margaret and nephew Paul. Their hand-holding got me through all this, and then some!

The award for *good sportsmanship* goes to Norman B. Rohrer, for permitting me to share the humorous anecdotes in chapter nine.

Awards for *generosity* go to everyone who paid for their books in advance. For a while, I was beginning to feel like the *Little Red Hen.* Then you came to my rescue and actually paid for the book *sight unseen*. How amazing!

Awards for *encouragement* go to all the thoughtful people who sent e-mails, letters and cards, telephoned, stopped by for a visit, or cooked suppers for me. I am truly grateful. Also, sincere thanks to each person who gave permission for me to use their name &/or quote their words.

Writing this book has not been an easy task. Besides spending hundreds of hours staring at a computer screen, I went through 7,500 sheets of paper and three laser toner cartridges.

I was telling a friend just the other day, "I used to have silver hair, now it's grey."

On the other hand, I can definitely recommend writing,

painting and other creative activities as excellent outlets for self-expression. I totally enjoyed the morning just before Christmas when Michaela and I painted pottery together. I'm very proud of my pale green ceramic mug with the bright yellow star—even if it does look like a five-year-old painted it!

My granddaughter Hayley (who is eight, going on thirty) seems to have everything in absolute perspective. While sitting with me after school recently, she said, "Grandma, I'm really lucky. I have a mom who's a hairdresser, a dad who can fix really big trucks, an uncle who's a movie star, an auntie who's a clown and a grandma who writes books."

God bless her, she's so good for me!

She also has this grand theory about life and skin. Just the other day she asked me, "Grandma, did you know that everyone has six skins?"

I smiled and asked her to explain.

"Well," she said cheerily. "First of all you have baby skin, then child skin, then teenage skin, then adult skin, then grandma skin, then nana skin—and then you die and go to heaven."

Those few words of wisdom from an eight-year-old really got me thinking—I only have one skin left. I'd better make good use of it!

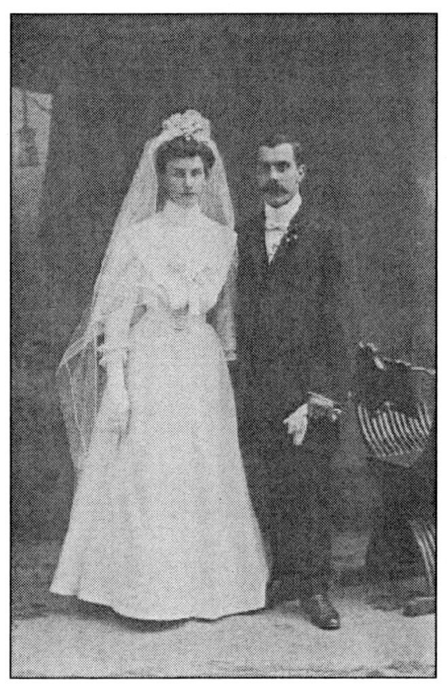

Pauline's paternal grandparents Anna Hollanwager married Arthur Ellis Johnson in 1907 in Luzern, Switzerland. Arthur was a professional photographer.

Pauline's grandfather, William Charles Raines and grandmother, Alice Beatrice Raines, with their three daughters, Dorothy (standing), Pauline's mother, Cecilia (seated), and infant Bertha (Auntie Bee). This photo was taken in 1916, when Grandpa Raines was about thirty. It is the only photograph we have of our mother as a young girl.

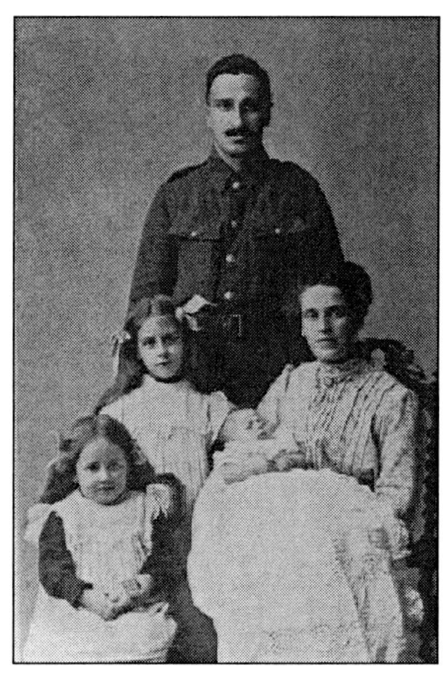

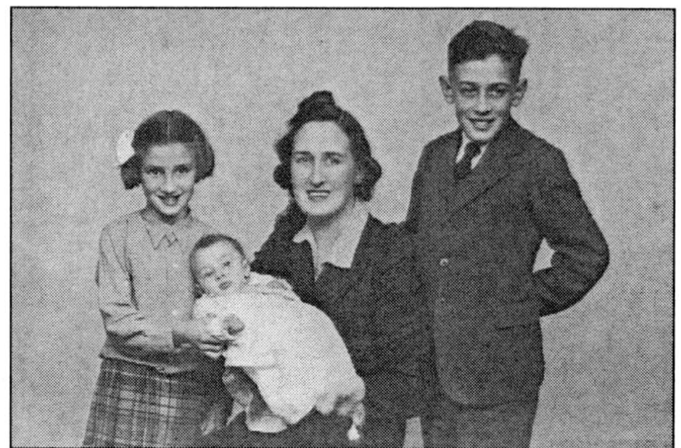

A 1945 family portrait. (L-R) Pat, our mother, Cecilia (holding infant Pauline), and David.

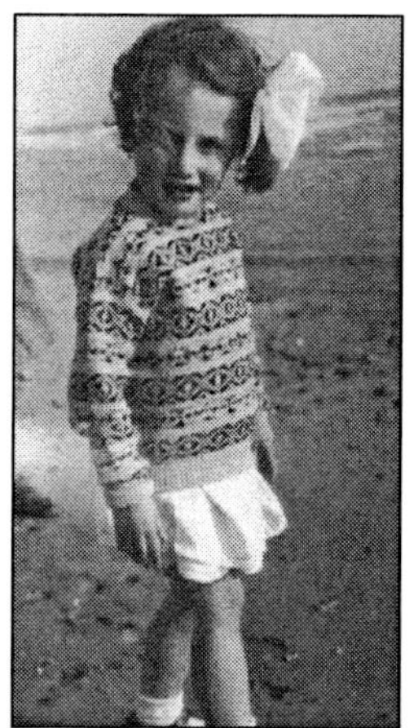

Pauline, age two, walking on Bournemouth Beach in England.

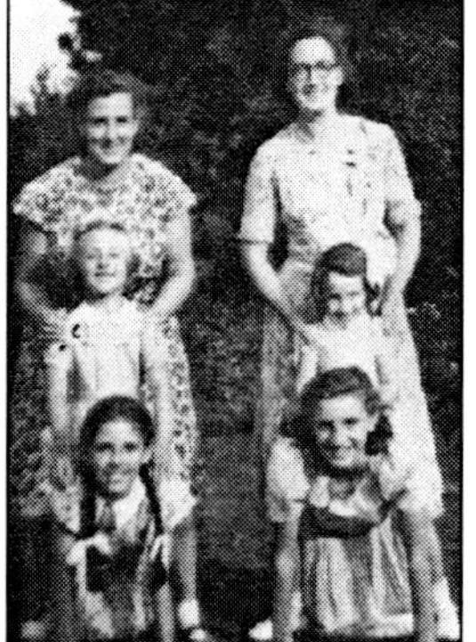

Here is a fun photo of sisters and cousins. On the left are Auntie Dorothy, Susan and Margaret. On the right are Cecilia, Pauline and Pat.

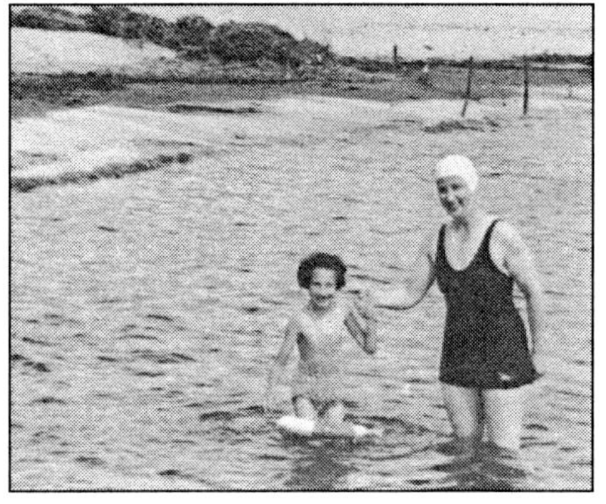

Swimming lessons for Pauline with Auntie Bee at Mudeford Beach near Bournemouth, 1953.

Walking down to the beach at Boscombe, which is 1-1/2 miles east of Bournemouth, in the summer of 1953. (L-R) Pat, Auntie Bee, Pauline and Grandma Raines.

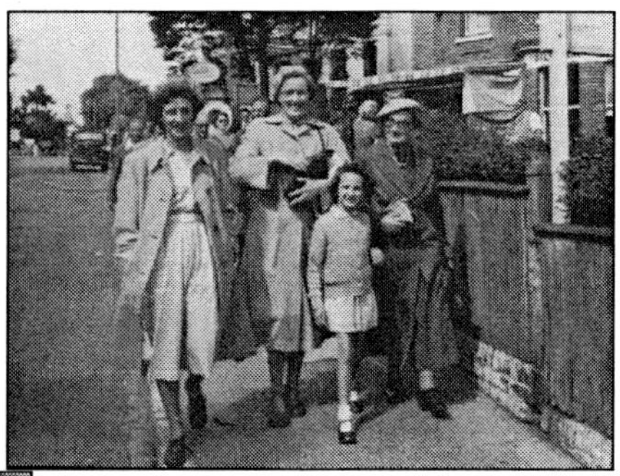

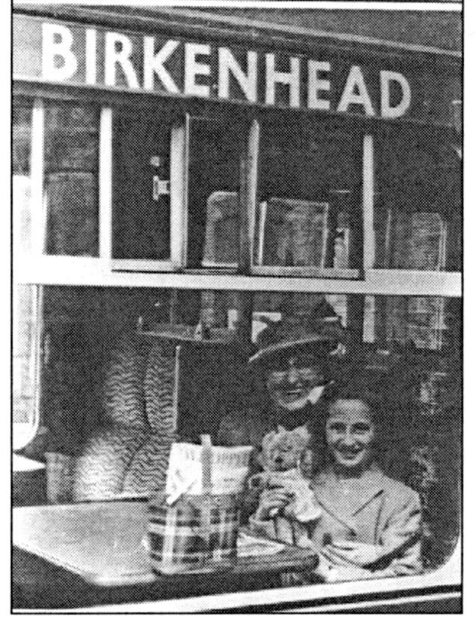

Auntie Bee and Pauline headed back to London by train. Circa: Easter 1954.

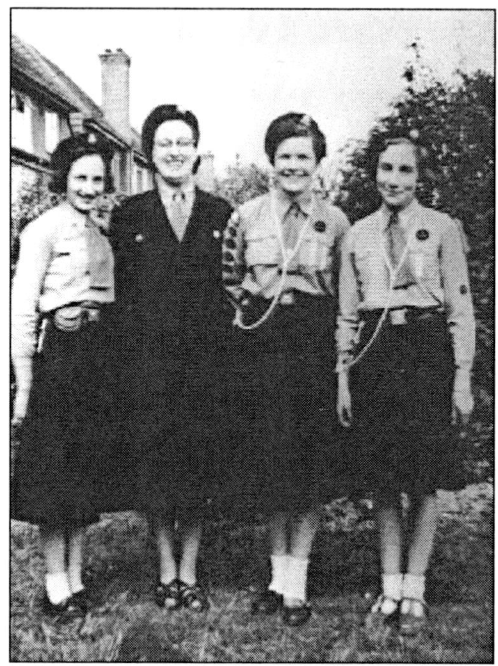

Girl Guides together, in the back yard of our house in West Drayton, Middlesex, England. (L-R) Pauline, Auntie Bee, Vera and Rosemary Hall. 1957.

Outside David and Margaret's house in Kinson. (L-R) David (holding infant Christine), Margaret, Paul and Pauline in 1959.

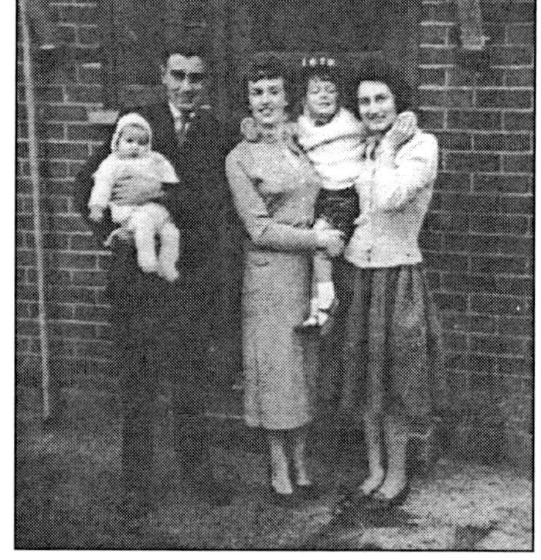

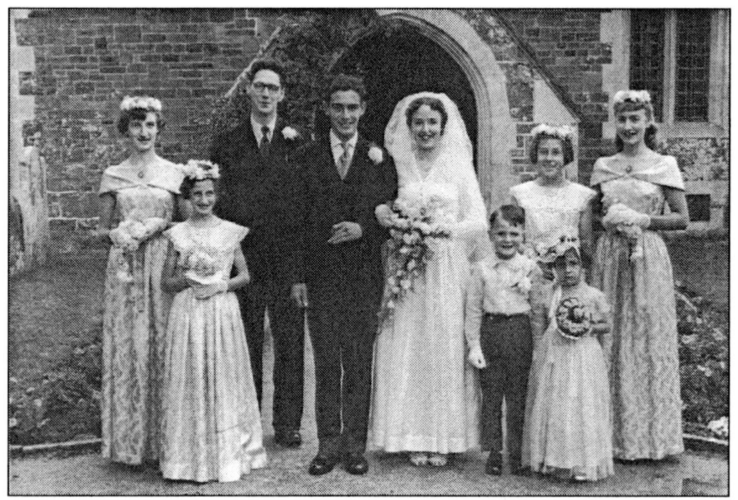

David and Margaret's wedding day, Sept. 4, 1954. (L-R) Pat, Pauline, Doug (best man), David, Margaret, Peter (Margaret's nephew), Susan (Pauline's cousin), Gwendoline (Margaret's niece) and Hazel (Margaret's friend).

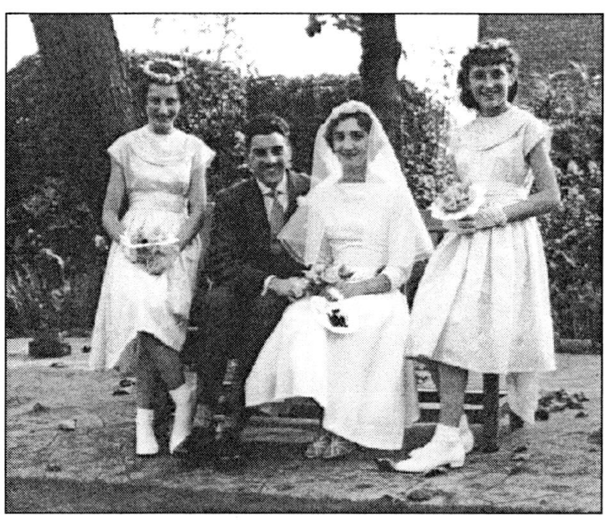

Pat and Jack's wedding day, Oct. 12, 1957. (L-R) Pauline, Jack, Pat and Susan (Jack's niece).

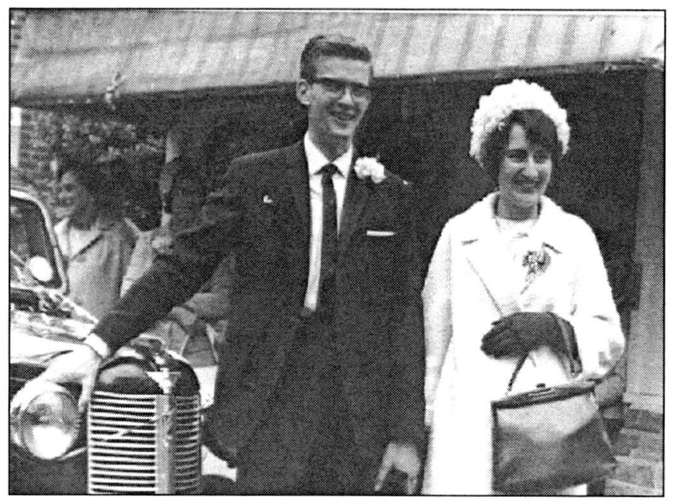

Martin and Pauline leaving for honeymoon- June 12, 1965.

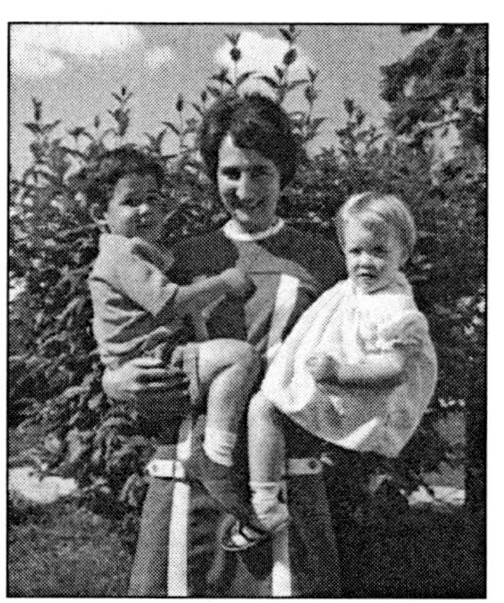

Pauline holding Elliot and Michaela- Carstairs, Alberta, July 1972.

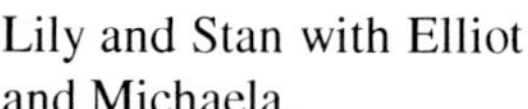

Lily and Stan with Elliot and Michaela.

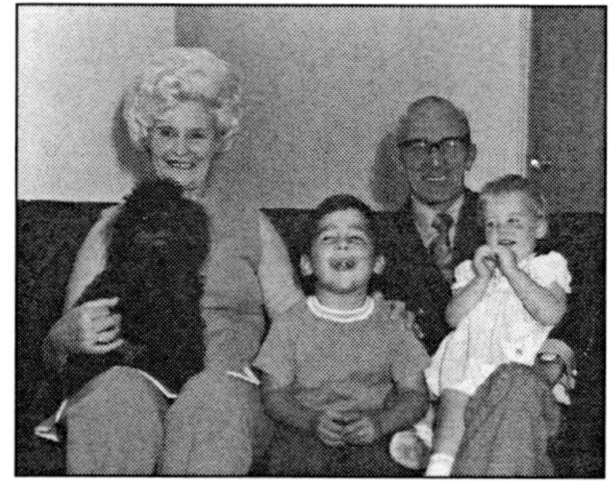

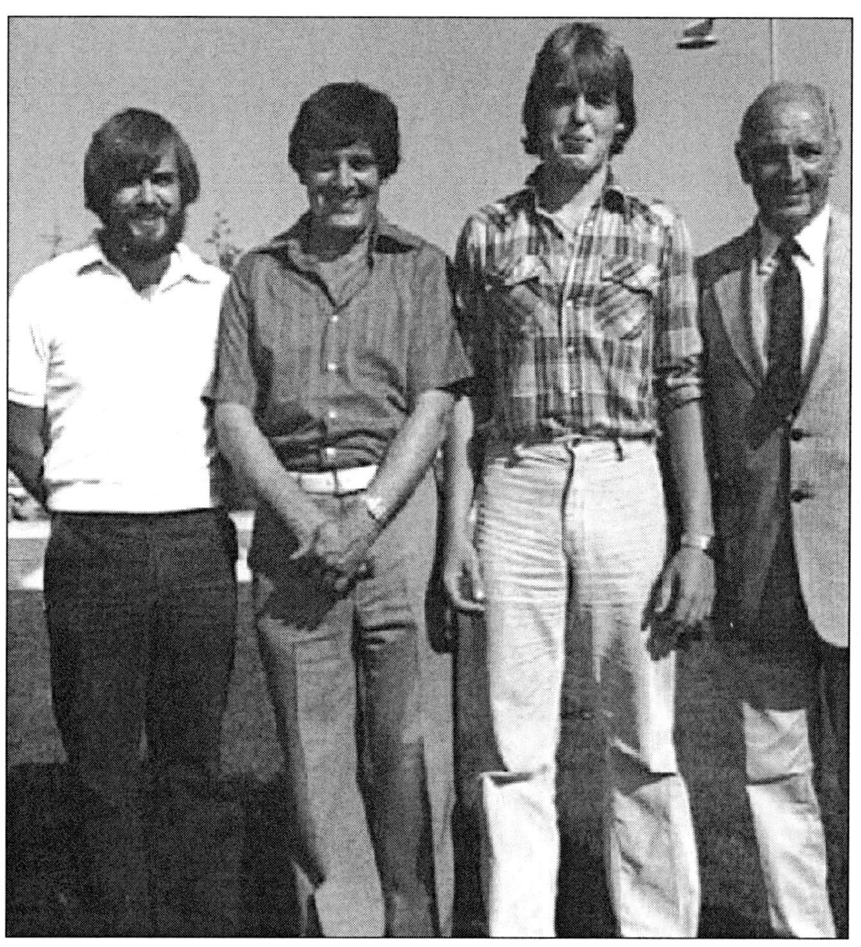

Three generations of Johnson men. (L-R) Paul, David, Stephen and Dad at the Vancouver Airport, October 1980.

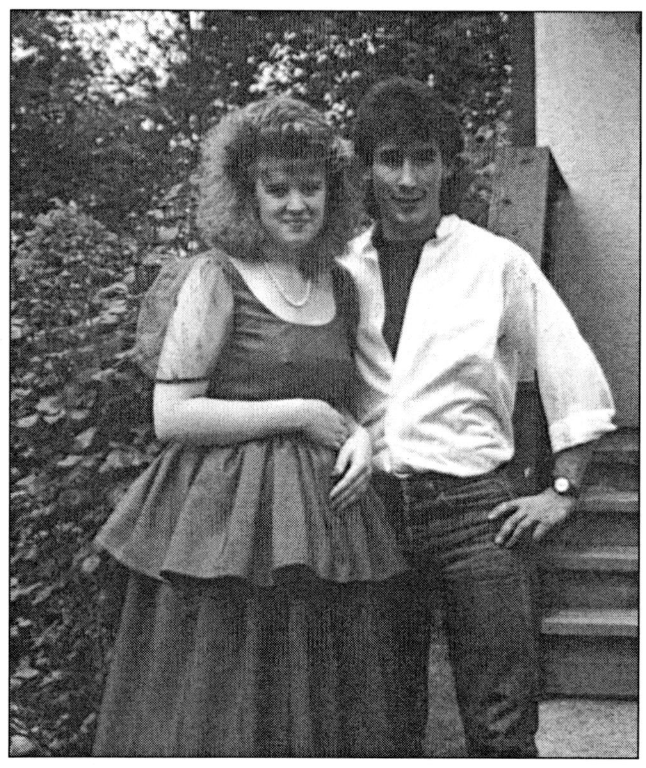

A grown-up Elliot and Michaela outside of our townhouse in Port Moody. Taken on Michaela's graduation from Grade 12 in June 1988.

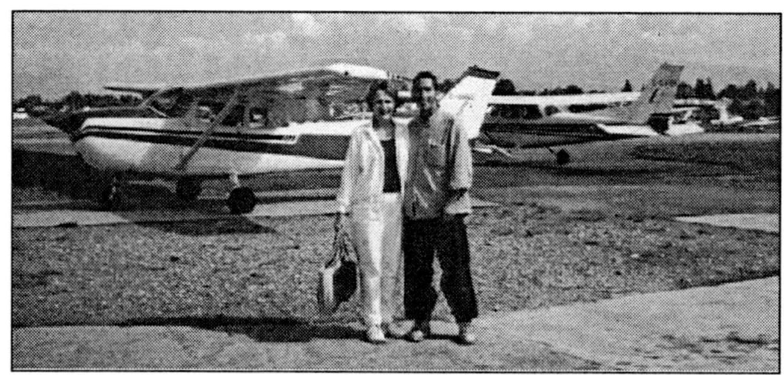

The day Elliot flew me to Victoria (I was much too proud of my son to be frightened!) September 1990

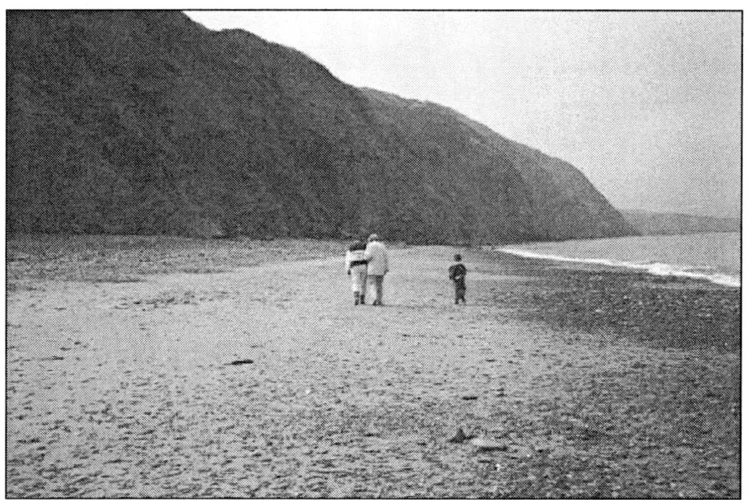

A stroll along the seashore at Aberaeron, Wales in May 1990. (L-R) Sally, Pat and my sister's grandson, James.

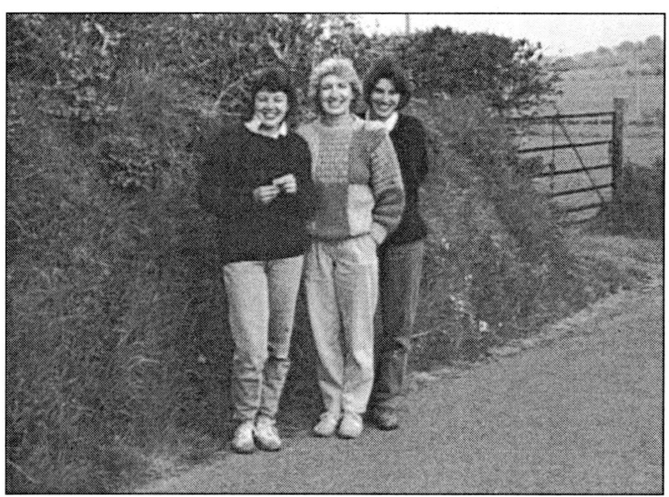

Walking down a country lane close to Pauline's niece, Sally's home at Dihewyd, Wales. (L-R) Sally, Pat and Maryjane.

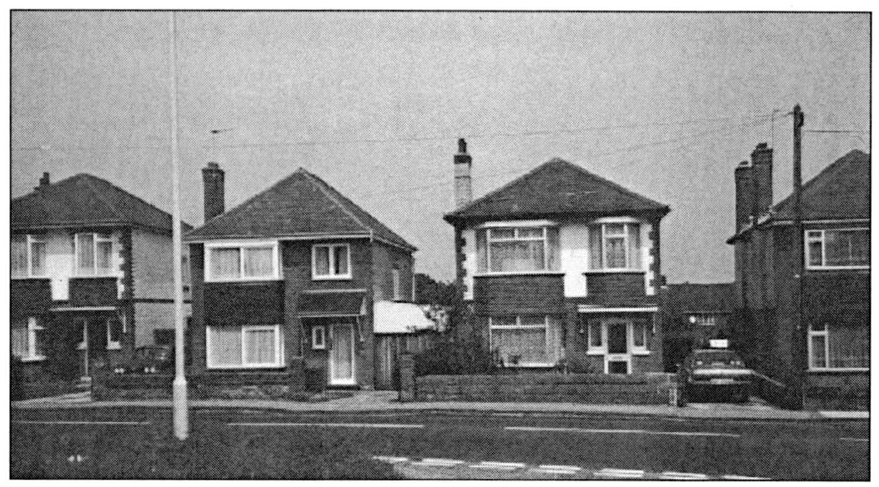

Here is a photograph of the house in Kinson where Pauline spent her teen years. Center-left is David and Margaret's house and center-right is Lily and Stan's house.

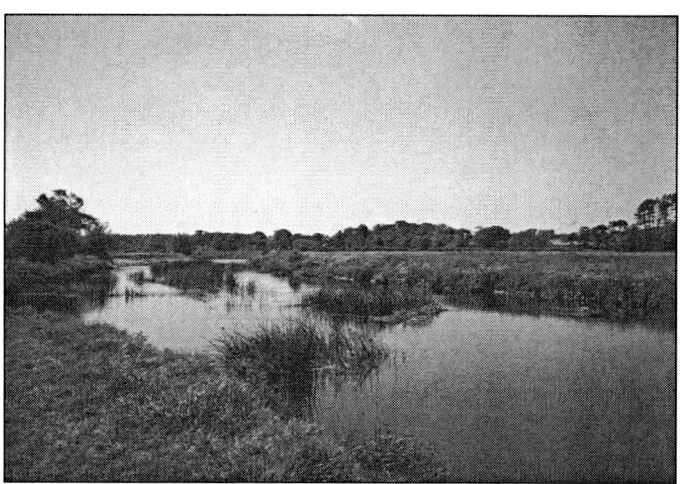

This is a view of the River Stour taken while I was on vacation in May 1990.

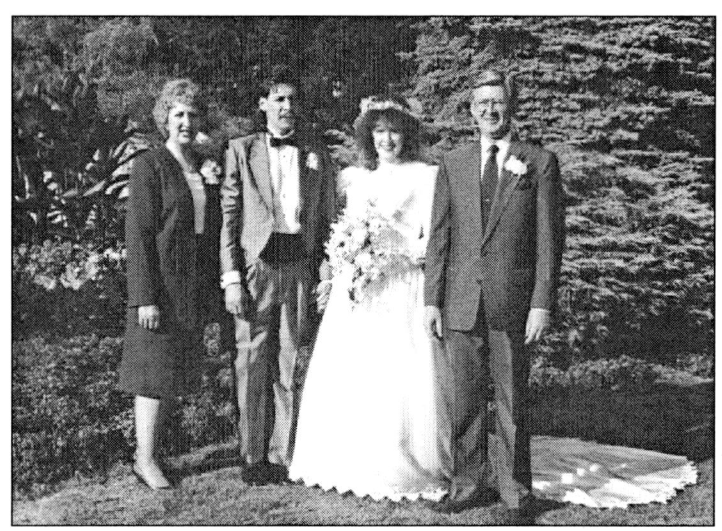

(L-R) Pauline, Frank and Michaela on their wedding day, and Martin. October 5, 1991.

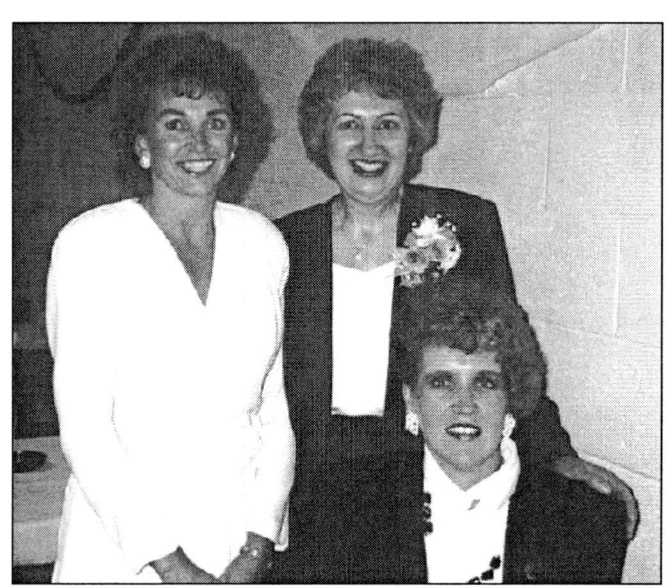

(L-R) Donna, Pauline and Kaye at Michaela and Frank's wedding. October 5, 1991

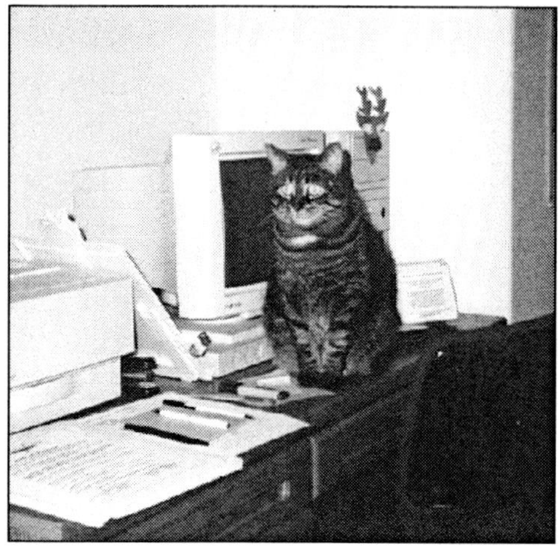

Curious “Mitzi” checks out the view from my computer desk.

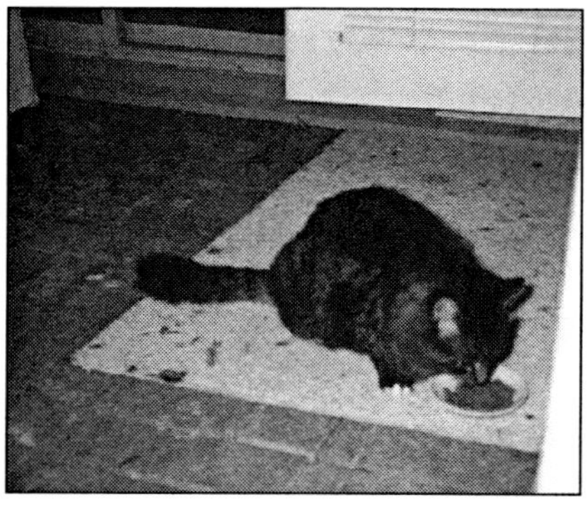

The ever-hungry Sterling munching on breakfast.

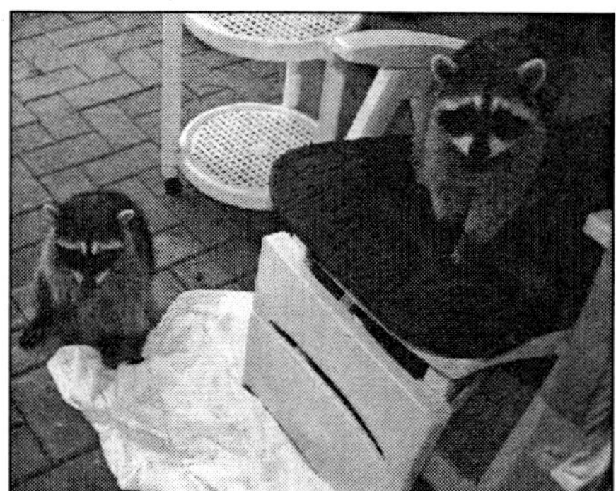

Those pesky raccoons ripped the blanket off Sterling’s patio chair again.

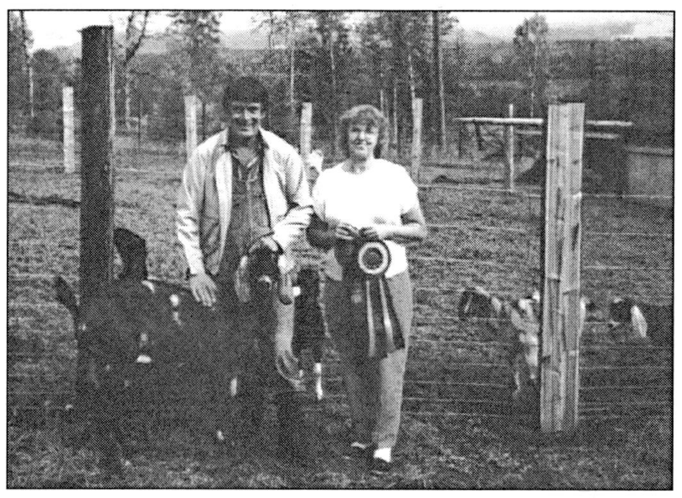

David and Margaret with prize-winning goats, September 1995.

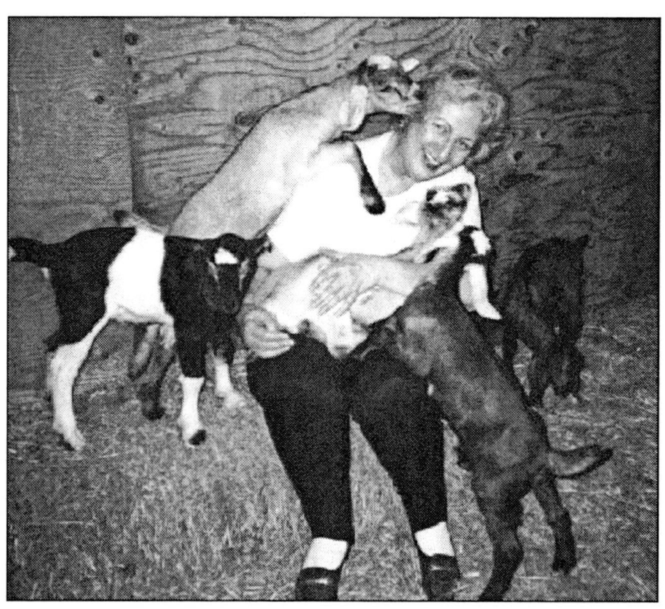

Pauline being attacked? By baby goats at Sorrento, BC. August 1995

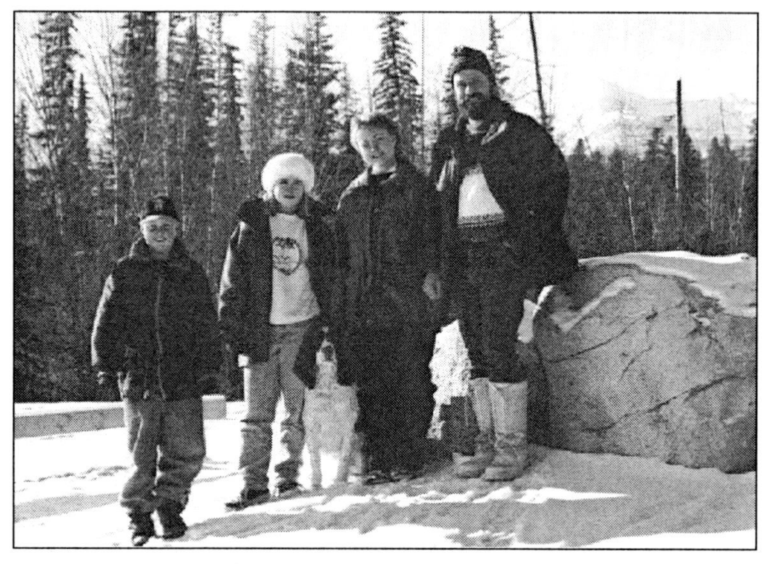

(R-L) Pauline's nephew, Paul with his wife, Laura, daughter, Amy and son, Brian. The photo was taken near their home in Valemount, BC December 1996.

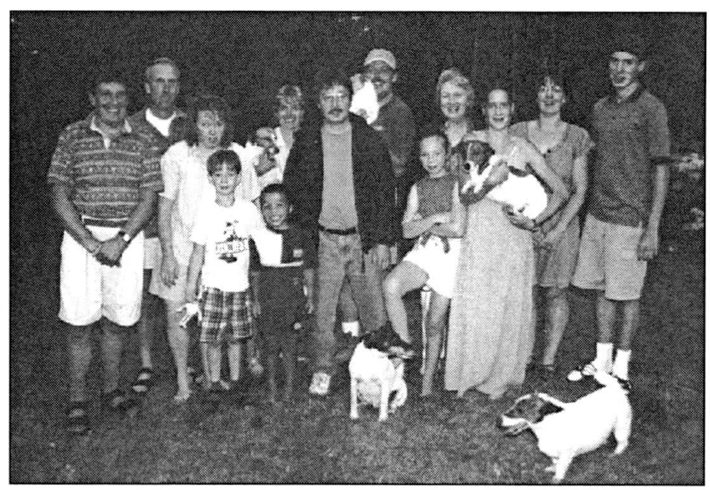

A family group photo taken by Margaret at Sorrento. (L-R) David, Rolfe, Brenda, Christopher, Ryan, Robin, Steve, Stephen J., Jennifer, Pauline, Angela, Christine, Greg and the dogs. August 1999

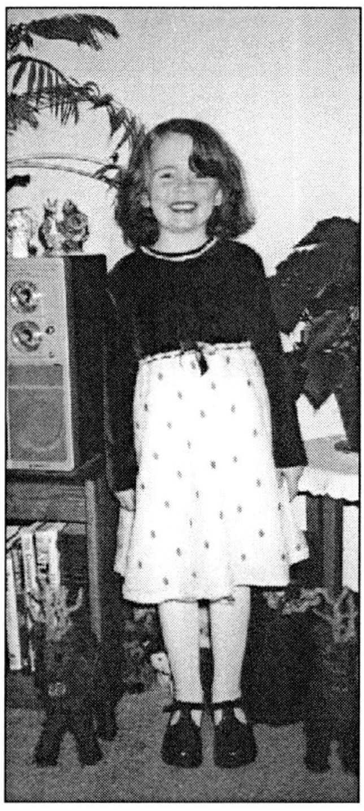

Hayley at Grandma's place, Christmas 1999

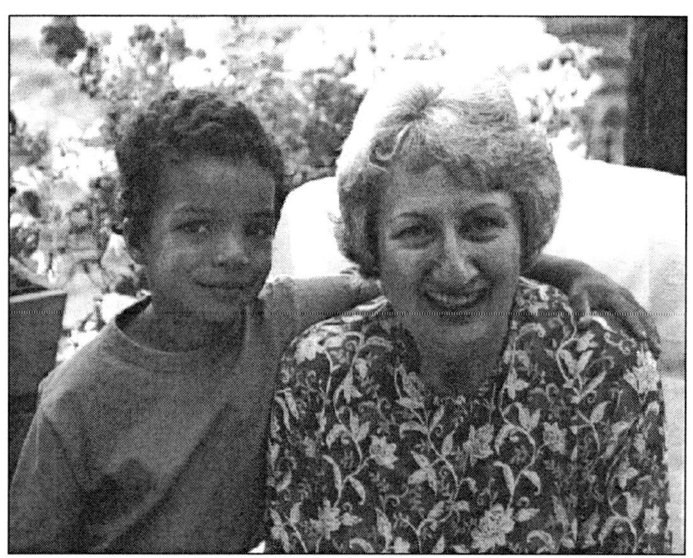

Stephen and Robin's son, Ryan, with Auntie Pauline at Sorrento, BC August 2000

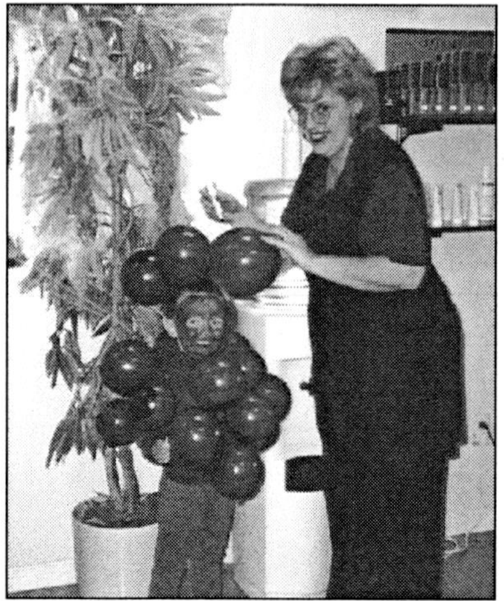

Hayley being 'made up' as a bunch of grapes by Mom, Michaela, October 2000

Little Maxwell, Elliot and Grandma Pauline, November 2000.

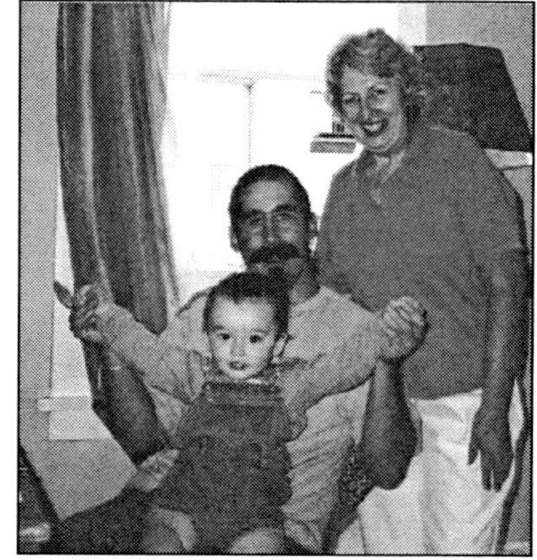

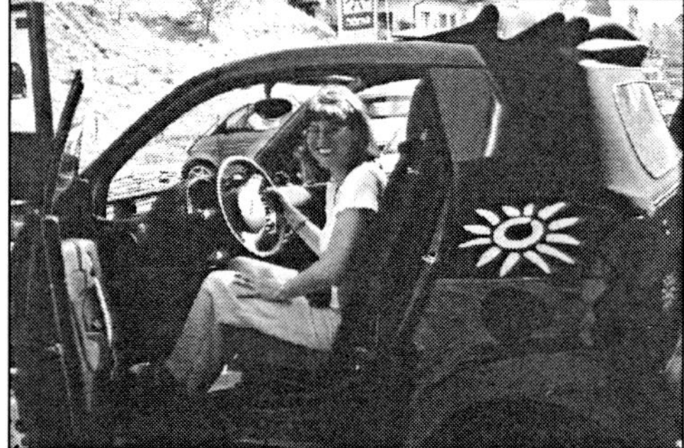

Pauline's niece, Maryjane, test-driving a 'smart car' in Luzern, Switzerland.
Sep. 2000.

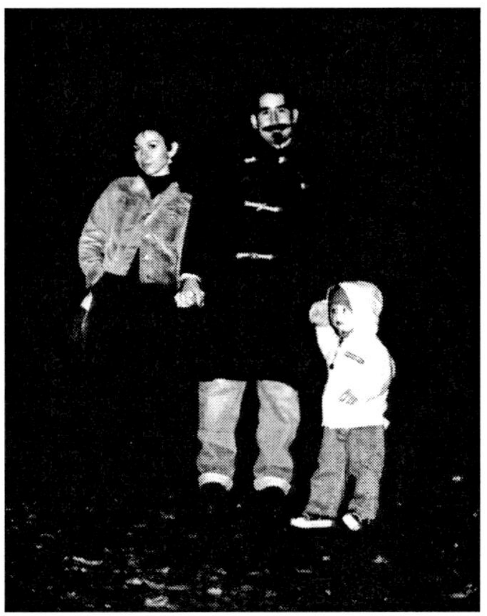

Gosia, Elliot and Maxwell at Cates Park in North Vancouver.

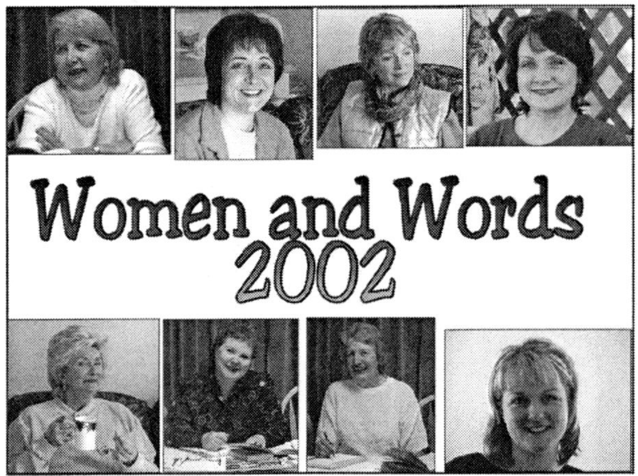

Women and Words Writers' Group 2002. (L-R) Ann, Carmen, Halia, Jacquie, Lillian (honorary member), Lyn, Pauline, Tara (Photo creation by Lyn Ayre www.ayresdigitaldoodlings.com)

ISBN 155369223-3
9 781553 692232